T0129393

*Vibrational Healing through the Chakras*

OTHER BOOKS BY JOY GARDNER, AKA JOY GARDNER-GORDON

*Death by Email* (Vibrational Healing Productions, 2001)

*Pocket Guide to Chakras* (The Crossing Press, 1998)

*Body/Mind Journeys* (Vibrational Healing Productions, 1995)

*The Healing Voice: Traditional & Contemporary Toning,
Chanting & Singing* (The Crossing Press, 1993)

*Our Earth Journey* (The Crossing Press, 1991)

*The New Healing Yourself* (The Crossing Press, 1989)

*Color and Crystals: A Journey Through the Chakras*
(The Crossing Press, 1988)

*Tantra and Brown Rice* (Healing Yourself Press, 1988)

*Healing Yourself During Pregnancy* (The Crossing Press, 1987)

*A Difficult Decision: A Compassionate Book About Abortion*
(The Crossing Press, 1986)

*The Book of Guidance* (Healing Yourself Press, 1985)

*Pink Tara: Teachings of the Heart from a Goddess of the New Age*
(Healing Yourself Press, 1985)

*Healing The Family* (Bantam Books, 1982)

*Healing Yourself* (Healing Yourself Press, 1972)

# VIBRATIONAL HEALING
## THROUGH THE CHAKRAS

*with Light, Color, Sound,*
*Crystals, and Aromatherapy*

JOY GARDNER

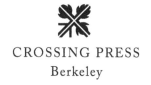

CROSSING PRESS
Berkeley

NOTE TO THE READER:
The names of clients mentioned herein have been changed to protect their privacy. In most cases places and specific facts related to these clients have been changed, and in some instances their stories are the blending of two or more actual individuals. All the facts are true and accurate.

The remedies and techniques described herein are given as information, and not as a prescription. They have not been tested on a broad sample of individuals or scientifically established. Therefore, neither the author nor the publisher can take responsibility for any ill effects that may be produced as a result of using these remedies and techniques: the reader does so at his or her own risk.

Copyright © 2006 by Joy Gardner

All rights reserved. Published in the United States by Crossing Press, an imprint of the Crown Publishing Group, a division of Random House, Inc., New York.
www.crownpublishing.com
www.tenspeed.com

Crossing Press and the Crossing Press colophon are registered trademarks of Random House, Inc.

Library of Congress Cataloging-in-Publication Data
Gardner, Joy.
Vibrational healing through the charkas with light,
color, sound, crystals, and aromatherapy/Joy Gardner.
p. cm.
Included bibliographical references.
1. Chakras 2. Healing 3. Self-care. Health. I. Title
RZ999.G3 14 2005
615.8'5-dc22
2005049705

ISBN-13 978-1-58091-166-5

Cover design by Leslie Waltzer, Crowfoot Design
Text design by Tasha Hall
Production work on illustrations on pages 53, 56, 60, and 66 by Akiko Shurtleff.
Illustrations on pages 53, 56, 60, and 66 copyrighted by Joy Gardner.

First Edition

146119709

# DEDICATION

*To two beloved mentors—*

*Elisabeth Kubler-Ross (1926–2004)*
*and*
*Kumu Hula Raylene Ha'alelea Kawaiae'a*

*Your gifts are too great to describe.*

# Contents

# Invocation and Gratitude

HEAVENLY FATHER, EARTHLY MOTHER, THOSE OF YOU IN THE Plant, Animal, and Mineral Kingdoms, beloved Angels and Elementals, and my own High, Middle, and Lower Selves, thank you for assisting me in all that I do. Bless this book and all who read it.

I give thanks to my clients and students, particularly those who were receptive to my early explorations into uncharted territories. Your faith in me and your feedback have been invaluable.

Thanks to my dear friend, Jonathan Mather, N.D., for helping me brainstorm and fine-tune the Spectrum of Biological Frequencies. Karen McDaniel, *mahalo* for your editorial and loving support and dedication throughout the creation of this book. Angela Rosa, R.N., thanks for your invaluable help with the aromatherapy section. Marya Grosse, N.P., thanks for reading the manuscript and for your great feedback.

Appreciation to Dr. Valerie Hunt and Bruce Tainio for your innovative research. Special kudos to my highly competent and supportive editorial team at Crossing/Ten Speed Press, including Jo Ann Deck, Carrie Rodrigues, and Judith Dunham.

And to my readers: Without you this book would not be possible.

All My Relations.

*A Hui Hou!*

# Introduction

Each child has at birth, a Bowl of perfect Light. If he tends his Light, it will grow in strength, and he can do all things—swim with the shark, fly with the birds, know and understand all things. If, however, he becomes envious or jealous, he drops a stone into his Bowl of Light, and some of the Light goes out. Light and the stone cannot hold the same space. If he continues to put stones in the Bowl of Light, the Light will go out, and he will become a stone. A stone does not grow, nor does it move. If at any time he tires of being a stone, all he needs to do is turn the bowl upside down, and the stones will fall away, and the Light will grow once more.—*Tales from the Night Rainbow*[1]

WE ARE ALL VIBRATIONS. THERE IS A HARMONIC FREQUENCY TO which all life is attuned. The human body is made up of frequencies that form a harmonic and balanced whole when a person is

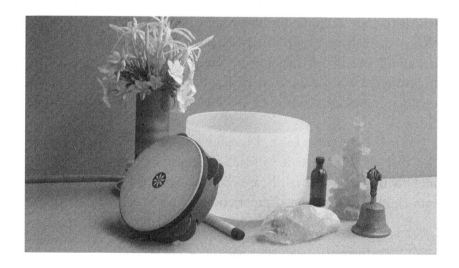

healthy. The vibrations of the body easily go out of tune when a person experiences physical or emotional stress. Vibrational healing employs vibratory tools to help the body remember its own healthy harmonic resonance. Once the body is in balance, it can fight off harmful organisms.

There are many vibratory tools. The primary ones that I use and discuss in this book include light and color (chromotherapy), crystals, aromatherapy, and sound. Other vibratory tools not covered in this book include flower remedies, gem elixirs, and homeopathy. You will find a glossary in the back of this book that contains definitions for these terms and other uncommon words found in this book.

It is difficult to conceptualize exactly how any form of energy healing actually works. There are many theories, and I will present the ones that seem most accurate to me, based upon my own experience.

In these busy times, few people can read a book from cover-to-cover. *Vibrational Healing through the Chakras* is divided into parts, each of which stands alone. You can read the table of contents to find subjects that match your areas of interest.

*Chakra* is a Sanskrit term that means "wheel" or "vortex." The chakras are nonphysical centers of spinning energy located in the energy field at the spine and other parts of the body. The human energy field, or aura, is a reflection of the combined frequencies of the chakras.

Most illness is characterized by blockage in the channels, which include acupuncture meridians, nerves, arteries, and veins. When there is blockage in any of these channels, inflammation, irritation, and illness may occur. The vibratory energies emanating from color, crystals, aromatherapy, light, and sound can break up these blockages, releasing the energy and allowing it to flow freely.

When I use these tools, I combine them with various modalities that allow my client to reach a deeper understanding of the underlying cause of her disease. Sometimes I will guide her back into childhood or prenatal experiences, or into past lives to explore the origins of her illness. I may help her to release emotions that have been repressed. I may guide her to examine dysfunctional core beliefs formed at an early age that still linger in her subconscious. In a future book, I will describe this work with core beliefs and underlying cause and how to do past life regressions.

Experiments with Kirlian photography (see Glossary) indicate that illness can be observed in the chakras *before* it manifests as physical disease. This means that a trained practitioner can detect energetic imbalances—and correct them—before they manifest as physical illness. This is best done through seasonal visits, ideally four times a year, and when there is significant stress in one's life.

In 1989, scientist Valerie Hunt proclaimed in her book, *Infinite Mind, Science of the Human Vibrations of Consciousness*, "In the future, it should be possible to diagnose field disturbances and to treat them months or even years before they are manifested in the physical tissue."[2] That future is now.

When the chakras come into balance, the body resumes its natural harmonic resonance, and illness does not manifest—or, if it is already present, symptoms disappear and generally do not return because the underlying cause of imbalance has been removed.

This book explains how to use the chakra system to detect imbalance, and how to bring the frequencies of light, color, sound, crystals, and aromatherapy through the chakras to restore harmony to the body, mind, emotions, and spirit. It traces the history, science, and traditional uses of Vibrational Healing in various cultures. It also describes my methods of Chakra Diagnosis and Vibrational Alignment™. And it introduces my new Spectrum of Biological Frequencies that gives specific numerical values for the frequencies of color, light, sounds, foods, herbs, and essential oils.

The vibratory tools can be used independently or in conjunction with other forms of energy work and bodywork, as well as conventional medicine, including psychiatry, psychology, and dentistry. This book is for people who wish to use Vibrational Healing for their own health and for those who are or wish to become practitioners of this healing art. It is for both beginning and accomplished healers. You will find that when you combine the vibratory tools with other forms of healing, the work becomes profoundly penetrating and goes from two to twenty times faster.

You may be able to free yourself from dependency upon chemical drugs and invasive surgical procedures that have potentially harmful side effects. We are fortunate to have a complete arsenal of heavy artillery medicine at our disposal. Doctors with drugs and surgical procedures can be angels of light when desperate situations arise. But there is no excuse for using a dagger to remove a splinter. There are usually gentler ways to bring your frequencies into balance and restore health.

In many parts of Europe today, where complementary medicine has long been practiced and appreciated, aromatherapists, herbalists, midwives, and other holistic practitioners are well respected and work side-by-side with allopathic physicians. In Switzerland, for example, homeopathy and kinesiology are covered by medical insurance. In the United States these healing arts are still considered by many to be questionable.

As of this date, crystal healing is still considered superstitious, despite the fact that crystals are being used universally in computers, clocks, lasers, and virtually all modern technology. The concept of healing with color is still viewed with skepticism, despite the fact that prisons have used pink holding rooms to quiet prisoners, and restaurants use orange décor to lure in customers.

Yet the times are changing. An article in the September 27, 2004 issue of *Newsweek* states that the federal government will spend $16 million on mind-body research in 2005, and private foundations will spend millions more. Acupuncture and massage are covered by some insurance plans in the United States and the Health Insurance Plan of New York, HIP USA, covers mind-body practices. Hospitals have mind-body clinics, and yoga classes are becoming widespread. Aromatherapy articles are appearing in popular women's magazines. According to a recent government survey, nearly half of all Americans used mind-body interventions in 2002.[3] The future holds the promise of truly complementary medicine.

Vibrations. What are they? We think of them as waves. I am sitting at a point that juts out into the ocean, on an island in Hawaii. The weather has been rough, the surf tossed by wind. The waves are variable and magnificent.

Sometimes they come rolling onshore in one long line, almost diagonal to the land, where they unfurl and crash against the wall of volcanic rock. Other times both ends roll while the center lags behind, dissolving into a blotch of foam. To my right, the distance of a football field out to sea, little waves are frolicking, almost perpendicular to the land, like a roller coaster of wavelets.

We take for granted the magnificent orchestration of sound and movement in every living form (though these sounds may be inaudible to our limited hearing and the movements may be invisible to our limited sight). Yet few among us do not thrill at the crash and thunder of waves against the rocks.

Here on my point, where waves move in a crazy array of parallel, diagonal, and perpendicular patterns, there is a subtle organization. It is as if a Grand Conductor was pointing her baton, beckoning some waves to enter now and telling others to wait a moment before crashing in, then telling yet another set to roll in slowly while the first set thunders dramatically against the cliffs. There is an exquisite periodicity, a perfect pulse, a harmonic metronome that puts all of life in order and makes it look and sound harmonious and pleasing to our eyes and ears—even in the worst tempest.

Bringing the macrocosm to the microcosm, you can observe the ocean of your own physical and energetic bodies, with at least an equal number and variety of vibrational patterns. But how much more susceptible these inner vibrations are to disruption!

By eating foods that wreak havoc in your belly and then subjecting yourself to a stressful argument, you set up antagonistic waves that come crashing through your body at a furious pace, creating a deafening and disharmonious roar that can literally be heard in your belly.

We know that when water pounds up against a cliff, it makes a huge roar. What if something prevents the water from making that sound? Can you imagine that the consciousness of that wave would carry around a sense of frustration and a lack of fulfillment until it is set free to express that roar?

When a person experiences a profound shock (such as the death of a loved one) it sets up an energy pattern that virtually demands to be expressed—like the sound of Navajo women keening when their men were killed in battle.

But most of us cut ourselves off from such raw forms of self-expression. Yet the unexpressed sound or vibration that should accompany the original shock remains trapped and stalks inside us, disrupting the normal flow of energies throughout the physical and energetic bodies.

Vibrational Healing combined with Underlying Cause and Emotional Release provides the context and opportunity to express old emotions that were stuffed and to release vibrations that may have evolved into vibratory disease signatures, enabling the natural rhythms of the body to return to their healthy harmonic frequency.

You can maintain the perfect rhythms that the Divine Conductor established within your body, or you can act—or allow others to act—as Grand Disrupters.

It is my hope that reading this book will inspire you to embrace new ways of thinking about your relationship with all of life; that you will begin to see yourself as a vibrating being in energetic interchange with your environment; giving and receiving energy from spirit and nature as well as other people, animals, and even unseen beings.

*Joy Gardner, Paia, Maui, Hawaii, 2005*

# Preface

I HAVE BEEN A HEALTH CARE PROFESSIONAL SINCE 1970, AND a Vibrational Healer since 1985, with thousands of students and clients throughout the United States, Canada, Europe, and Australia.

In the early 1970s, I worked as an herbalist and women's paramedic at the Country Doctor Community Clinic in Seattle. The clinic sponsored the first printing of my book, *Healing Yourself,* which was one of the first medicinal herbals in North America in modern times.

I had a recurrent cyst on my ovary, and though I knew how to make it shrink with herbs and fasting, I wanted a more permanent solution. British healer Rev. Helena Ram guided me through a series of spiritual journeys in which I met my Spirit Guides, worked with color, experienced past lives, and visualized myself inside my body. I made myself small, went into my ovaries, spoke to them, and derived profound insights about the underlying emotional causes of the cyst.

As Helena helped me express and clear away deep feelings that had been repressed since early childhood, I felt a profound change. Suddenly illness was no longer an enemy that had to be defeated, cut, burned, or poisoned. It was a teacher, a bringer of wisdom. Illness was the tip of the iceberg that gave crucial warning of a mass of unfinished business hidden just below the surface of conscious awareness.

After several sessions, I learned to guide others through Spiritual Journeys, and became far more than a physical healer. Being able to assist my clients to find the underlying cause of their ailments was endlessly fascinating. No two people were the same; every journey was unique.

As I continued to explore my hidden realms, I discovered a huge mass of unexpressed grief. Growing up with a bipolar mother, I learned early how to stuff my emotions and close down, to protect myself against her devastating mood swings. At age thirteen I experienced the loss of my only brother, my defender, who took his own life when he was nineteen. I had no idea how to cry or express my deep pain. Later, in my midtwenties, between the births of my two sons, I had a baby girl who died in utero just before she was born. Again, I ran away from my feelings. I left my husband and moved to Canda.

In 1978, I had the opportunity to attend a lecture by Swiss psychiatrist Elisabeth Kubler-Ross (1926–2004). During the 1970s Americans were in denial about death, and one rarely saw movies or TV programs in which people died. This diminutive, humble woman single-handedly made a huge contribution toward helping Americans overcome their fear of death.

I attended two of her five-day workshops, where I could finally give vent to the pain and grief that had so long been repressed. Then I went to Elisabeth's center, Shanti Nilaya, in Escondido, California, where I immersed myself in her work. I learned the skills of a death and loss counselor, which I brought back to British Columbia. There I helped start the Nelson and District Hospice Society, where I trained volunteers, and taught workshops on death and loss.

My thirst to explore new horizons as a healer brought me to Katrina Raphaell's books on crystal healing. When I read about the loving energies that rose quartz reputedly embodied, I wondered if this stone could help my client Theresa (a fictitious name) who lost her beloved in a rafting accident. His body was never recovered, and Theresa's grief was intense and prolonged. She could never be certain that someday he would not come walking in the door. Theresa and I made good progress during our sessions, but she could not break down and cry.

I purchased a large hunk of rose quartz, and when Theresa arrived for her next session, I tentatively inquired if she would lie down on the couch and let me put this big pink rock on her chest. She was amenable. Within seconds I watched with amazement as tears came streaming down her cheeks.

After that, the stones came rapidly into my life. I found a blue-and-green stone called azurite-malachite. When placed at the throat, the blue azurite seemed to stimulate the voice box, enabling clients to speak more openly, and the green malachite seemed to help them get in touch with their emotions. A striated pink stone called kunzite worked well to soften physical and emotional block-ages. A translucent brown stone called smoky quartz seemed to remove negativity from the body and from physical rooms. These stones quickly became an indispensable part of my healing practice.

Later I will tell about how chakras, sound, and aromatherapy came into my life and how I correlated the sounds and aromas with the chakras. My career as a sound healer was shaped by my work with Kubler-Ross, because my emphasis is upon making sounds for emotional release. I believe that toning is a universal language that bypasses the rational left brain and gives direct visceral emotional expression to the soul.

My first book on Vibrational Healing, *Color and Crystals—A Journey through the Chakras,* was published in 1988 when the word "chakra" was virtually unknown in the United States. To this date it has sold more than fifty thousand copies. Its initial success catapulted me into a position of authority in the field of healing with gemstones. The popularity of Shirley Maclaine's books during the eighties created a burgeoning interest in New Age books and crystals.

But during the early 1990s, Maclaine's popularity faded rapidly and many metaphysical bookstores and crystal shops closed down. In just a few months, my workshops on Crystal Healing plum-meted from seventy-five students to a mere five. I needed a new career.

So I went on retreat for three days of fasting, praying, and asking for Guidance. During that retreat I kept hearing the words, "Vibrational Healing." I had never heard that term before. I did not hear these words with my outer ears. It was more like a thought that came from a source outside myself. I called it "Guidance."

Until then, I considered myself a hopeless eclectic. I had too many interests and too many unrelated skills. During my three-day fast, when I heard the term Vibrational Healing, I began to realize that I could teach all my work with chakras, gemstones, sound, color, and aromatherapy under the umbrella of Vibrational Healing.

At first I thought my Death and Loss Workshop was completely separate. But a major part of death and loss work involves releasing old emotions so people can live fully in the present. When I am working on a client and I feel blockage in the emotional chakras, I often remove the stones from his body and encourage him to get up and grab a rubber hose and give vent to his anger—a technique I learned from Kubler-Ross. Once the anger and tears are released, there is an immediate opening, especially at the emotional second, third, and fourth chakras.

So my Death and Loss Workshop evolved into an Emotional Release Workshop. Within three days of my fast I structured a new program with a series of eight workshops that included all of the diverse work that I did for so many years.

The day after my fast I went to a bookstore and found the newly released book *Vibrational Medicine* by Richard Gerber, MD. I was amazed to find that Dr. Gerber used a similar term to describe the work that I was doing with color and gemstones at the chakras. This synchronicity felt like a strong confirmation of my guidance.

In 1989 I became the founder and director of the Vibrational Healing Program (see Resources). In 1995 I brought the workshops to the Big Island of Hawaii. For several years I also taught the program near Columbus, Ohio.

In October 2004, my grandson Keanu entered this world. In June 2005, I joined Keanu and my son and daughter-in-law on Maui.

# PART I

# VIBRATIONAL HEALING AND THE CHAKRAS

A TRUE UNDERSTANDING OF VIBRATORY ENERGY COULD LEAD TO the proverbial fountain of youth. The second law of thermodynamics states that all matter progresses from organization to disorganization and then to turmoil. For humans this means that as we get older we become progressively less coherent at a cellular level until we die.

However, Nobel biochemist Ilya Prigogine (1917–2003) discovered that when energy is introduced into any field, its complexity increases. Along with the complexity comes greater refinement, rather than entropy.[1] The vibratory tools of light, color, crystals, aromatherapy, and sound, pump energy into the cells, creating greater complexity and thereby increasing longevity.

The ultimate form of Vibrational Healing is to be in nature, charging your brain through the sunlight entering your eyes (especially when you remove your glasses, sunglasses, and contacts), and by the sounds entering your ears and the aromas entering your nostrils. It is especially rewarding if you can be in the presence of natural waveforms, such as moving water and wind.

Drinking water is essential for maintaining your electromagnetic balance. Kinesiologists (see Glossary) cannot get accurate readings if a person has not been drinking enough water because water ionizes salts and provides the optimum environment for efficient conduction of nerve impulses.[2][3] So be sure to drink plenty of pure water.

In the early 1970s, Dr. Valerie Hunt was teaching neurophysiology and psychology at UCLA. As a child she had a near-death experience, which may account for why she was so unusually open-minded for a professor of her era. Dr. Hunt developed a method for measuring the human energy field (see "Science of the Chakras" on page 24) and found that it would expand when people were in the mountains or near the sea. "If a person's field was particularly small, we would send him to the pool to swim or to a cold shower, or have him walk barefoot on the grass. . . These increased his field and improved his feelings. . ."[4]

Living in Hawaii near the ocean allows me to enjoy these natural waveforms on a daily basis. Even when I was a young woman, working as a secretary on the South Side of Chicago, I managed to go outside and walk on the tree-lined streets during lunch or coffee breaks. When I worked downtown, I walked to the Buckingham Fountain, to watch the dance of colored waters while I sat and ate my lunch.

In Masaru Emoto's beautiful book, *The Message from Water*, this Japanese researcher shows photographs of crystal patterns formed in frozen drops of water taken from different locations. Most of the water from relatively untouched natural settings forms exquisite crystalline patterns, whereas most water from polluted cities collapses in upon itself.

Even more remarkable, the water crystals seem to respond to emotions, words, music, and essential oils. Emoto exposed the water to heavy metal music, and it made an explosive pattern without crystal formations. When the water was exposed to the classical and highly symmetrical Bach's Goldberg Variations, it formed an exquisite geometrical crystal.

Emoto set a container of chamomile essential oil next to the water, and the water crystals formed into amazing crystalline facsimiles of chamomile flowers. The same thing happened with fennel oil.[5] Most of these photos can be seen at www.hado.com.

If the water in our bodies is that responsive to music and essential oils, this is clear evidence of the power of the vibratory tools.

Fabien Maman showed that our very cells respond directly to music. In 1974, while working as a professional jazz musician, he observed that certain musical keys would energize both the musicians and the audience. He brought this insight to French physicist Joel Sternheimer, who discovered that elementary particles vibrate in accordance with musical laws. Their combined research indicated that body tissues, organs, and acupuncture meridians each have a musical note.

Maman used Kirlian photography (see Glossary) to photograph the changes in the electromagnetic fields around healthy cells while playing a xylophone to them. He found that the slight difference of a half tone would produce a completely different shape and color in the energy field of the cell. When he played the note C, they became longer; D elicited a variety of colors, E caused them to become spherical, and A changed their color field from red to pink.

Maman took a sample of blood from a subject's finger and asked her to sing the seven notes of the major scale to her own blood cells. The cells' energy field changed with each note until she sang the note F, at which point the cells resonated perfectly with her voice, producing a balanced, round shape with vibrant magenta and turquoise colors. He concluded that this note was the *fundamental* sound of the singer, and that a person's fundamental sound, *produced by his or her own voice*, is the most powerful healing tool to harmonize and regenerate the body at the cellular level.[6]

## Physics and Metaphysics

During the twentieth century, science was a kind of god. Now we are experiencing a new way of perceiving the universe. It is a vast change that calls upon us to totally reconfigure the way we look at virtually everything.

The old paradigm is known as Newtonian physics. It presents us with a tidy universe in which Mother Nature performs like clockwork, predictably following laws that can be known and repeated. Scientists of the Newtonian era believed that the mysteries of the universe would all be revealed simply by examining increasingly smaller blocks of matter with increasingly sensitive lenses until eventually they would be able to explain how even consciousness evolved from matter.

Then quantum physics blew that whole worldview apart. The double slit experiment was used to determine whether a photon is a wave or a particle. It employs a screen with two narrow slits side by side, like a booth at the circus where you throw a sandbag through the holes. We know that one sandbag will go through one hole at a time. If the photon is a particle, it will go through just one slit, like the sandbag. If it is a wave, it will go through both slits.

Scientists found that sometimes an electron behaves like a particle and goes through just one slit, and other times it behaves like a wave, passing through both slits at once. Michael Talbot, author of *The Holographic Universe*, waxes poetic as he describes the behavior of such an electron: "You throw a pebble at a window and it either hits the window and bounces off or it breaks through. You shoot an electron at a barrier and it can hit, bounce off, it can stop just before the window, dematerialize, materialize on the other side, it can stop just before the window and reverse its direction. These electrons were behaving like shape-shifting shamans. The scientists had to conclude that subatomic particles are sometimes particles and sometimes waves, and they can instantly change from one to the other."[7]

The term *quantum* is used to describe something that possesses both particle and wave aspects. So *quantum theory* is a theory in physics based on the principle that matter and energy have the properties of both particles and waves. What appears to be solid is actually—at the atomic level—more than 99.9999 percent empty space! The protons and electrons are sometimes particles that can be measured (millions of times smaller than the tiniest atom) and sometimes waves of vibrating energy.[8]

To get a clear image of the size of subatomic particles, imagine a fourteen-story building turned sideways; this is the diameter of the dome of Saint Peter's basilica in the Vatican. Now imagine an atom that has been blown up to the size of this dome. How big would the nucleus of this atom be? The size of a grain of salt! And the electrons revolving around this grain of salt would be about two thousand times smaller, that is, the size of dust particles. But even a dust particle is a particle. According to quantum mechanics, subatomic particles should actually be called wave/particles because they are sometimes waves and sometimes particles that have "tendencies to exist."[9]

In the seemingly stable human body, 98 percent of the atoms are replaced in the period of just one year, according to radioisotope studies conducted at Oak Ridge laboratories in California. Your heart and brain cells are pretty durable, but your liver cells last only a few years, your red blood cells live for just two or three months, and your skeleton is recreated every three months. Most of your skin cells are replaced in just two weeks, and the cells of your stomach are replaced in only a few days.[10]

The implications of this are almost unfathomable. It's like giving a kid some blocks and telling him to erect a building. Then, after he has built a whole city, you tell him, "Those aren't really blocks. They're just a bunch of empty space with waves that are sometimes particles. We can't be sure they exist; all we know is they have tendencies to exist."

This could make a kid (or a Newtonian scientist) feel very insecure. But if you work with energy, and if you know from experience that seemingly miraculous healings do happen almost instantaneously, it can come as a great relief to have a way of explaining and understanding the reality you live in.

## Why Vibrational?

Hovering inside the doorway of our Santa Cruz, California home, my son and I held onto each other for dear life. It was 1989 and we were in the middle of the massive 7.2 Loma Prieta earthquake near Santa Cruz, California. It felt as if we were on a sailing ship, but instead of being tossed on the waves of the ocean, we watched in amazement as the very stuff of our living room turned into one big wave that undulated before our eyes. Kids out on the road lamented that they didn't have their surfboards because the pavement literally turned into a huge rolling wave.

If I ever doubted that solid substance is an illusion, I now had living proof. Scientists have a word for this phenomenon; they call it "liquefaction." We live in a reality made up of particles that can turn into waves. The concept of something that is sometimes matter and sometimes vibration is crucial to Vibrational Healing.

Allopathic doctors are trained in the old Newtonian scientific paradigm that conceives of the body as a machine that must obey the basic laws of nature. Quantum mechanics reveals a world of subatomic particles that do not obey the same laws. When the will aligns with the mind and spirit and when you can conceptualize the physical body as a highly amorphous entity, you can literally create your own reality. As you remove all mental and emotional obstacles, the body will leave behind all misalignment known as disease and naturally realign to its own healthy harmonic resonance.

With energetic forms of healing we acknowledge the profound role that the emotions play in directly influencing the balance or imbalance of the structures of the body. We also acknowledge the role of subtle forces and subtle fields, including love, touch, prayer, positive thinking, belief, and a desire to live.

The possibilities of using vibrational tools for health and healing are enormous. There are also possibilities for creating illness through the deliberate or inadvertent abuse of vibrational frequencies. For example, animals who graze under high-voltage power lines have stunted growth. Infants exposed to x-rays in utero have a 40 percent increased risk of childhood leukemia and a 50 percent increased risk of all other cancers.[11]

It has been rumored that diseases can be reproduced vibrationally as "disease signatures," which can then be sprayed in the air or delivered by way of chemtrails, using harmonics and subharmonics to make them more lethal and infectious.[12]

We know that certain vibrations create illness. Why is it so difficult to believe that vibrations can create health?

## Overview of Chakras and the Human Energy Field

Chakra is a Sanskrit word that means wheel or vortex. The chakras are nonphysical centers of spinning energy. The relative openness of the chakras governs a person's ability to receive and generate vibratory energy, known as *chi, prana*, and *mana* in China, India, and Hawaii, respectively.

The three chakras below the chest are called the lower chakras. Through these centers we receive and transmit sexual, emotional, and social energy. The heart is the middle chakra, through which we experience unconditional love. The three chakras above the chest are the higher chakras. Through these centers we receive and transmit psychic and spiritual energy.

There are seven levels of openness at each chakra. You must have at least one level of openness in each chakra to maintain life.[13] Most people have a moderate amount of openness at each chakra, with a higher degree of openness at one or two of them. Those who have the gift of clairvoyance explain that when a chakra is relatively closed, the color relating to that chakra becomes dim or obscure. When a chakra is completely open, the corresponding color predominates in that person's aura. When all the chakras are wide-open, the aura becomes white.

Of the many different chakra arrangements, I prefer the rainbow system, which identifies seven major chakras. When counting the chakras, most systems begin at the bottom and go to the top. Each of the seven major chakras is located in the vicinity of the spine, near a major nerve plexus, a major endocrine gland, and one or more internal organs. The chakras convert higher subtle energies into the cellular structure of the physical body, stepping down energy of one form and frequency to a lower level energy. This lower and more substantial energy is then translated into hormonal, physiologic, and ultimately cellular changes at the physical level.[14]

As an example of how this works, I have a client (I will call her Annette) who had Graves' disease, a form of hyperthyroidism in which the thyroid glands (located on either side of the Adam's apple in the neck) produce too much thyroid. This condition is believed to occur because of a blood defect in suppressor T lymphocytes, or T cells. Metaphorically, her blood lacked a certain kind of warrior cell that would normally hold the production of thyroxin in check.

Annette's doctor wanted to remove her thyroid gland surgically or destroy it with radioactive iodine, which is standard treatment for Graves' Disease. He warned her she would die if she did not follow one of these procedures.

When she came to see me, I did not encourage her to go against her doctor's advice. But Annette was determined to follow her own intuition, and I followed her lead. I do not cure diseases. I simply guide a client to explore what led to the imbalance, and then I support her in expressing, releasing, and resolving those issues. When I combine this work with the vibrational tools, most diseases improve or clear up quickly, particularly if the client is highly motivated. I believe that the healing (or lack of it) is the client's responsibility. Annette was a good example, as this story reveals.

I used my long thin crystal wand to feel the spin of energy at Annette's chakras, including the subchakras at each hip. The left hip holds the energy of the mother during the first three years of a child's life and prenatally, and the right hip holds the energy of the father during the same period.

As I felt the spin of energy at Annette's left hip I felt my awareness merge with the emotional body of Annette's mother while Annette was an infant. Her mother seemed preoccupied and unenthusiastic about being a mother. At Annette's right hip I felt for the energy of her father, but he was not present.

The energy of the other chakras was not remarkable until I came to her third chakra, the center of power and self-worth, which was distinctly weak. I placed a yellow citrine at her solar plexus. Her heart chakra felt normal.

When I came to the throat chakra I could feel an irregular energy. It felt jerky and thin. I put a drop of blue German chamomile oil at the hollow of her neck, which is calming and soothing. Then I placed a smooth round azurite-malachite stone at her throat. Green malachite stirs up the emotions and brings them to the surface; blue azurite stimulates the voice box so a person feels the impulse to speak about her emotions.

I told Annette what I perceived at each chakra, and she replied that she was the last of five children; she was the accident. Just before she was born, her father abandoned the family. "My mother was a basket case for years."

As a small child, Annette realized that the best way to get approval was by being perfectly quiet. She was rarely allowed to talk, and certainly could not sing or shout, or the punishment would be severe. Annette brought this repressive pattern into her adulthood. She was a docile and highly supportive woman who never contradicted anyone. "Everyone says that I'm very easy to get along with."

The thin feeling at Annette's throat came from her inability to express herself. The jerky feeling came from her suppressed emotions, as if they were chomping at the bit to be released.

I encouraged Annette to scream. I gave her an 18-inch length of heavy-duty industrial rubber hose, urging her to get in touch with her resentment and anger by hitting the mat with all her strength. She confided that before she came to see me, she made up her mind that her survival depended upon opening her throat and releasing her rage. Finally she found the courage to open her mouth, and she released forty-nine years of repressed fury.

It took only one session to bring her body back to normal. I believe that the azurite-malachite opened the door that allowed her to scream, which then allowed the energy to move through her throat chakra, stimulating her thyroid gland and causing the T cells to wake up and resume their function of blocking the excess production of thyroxine.

Annette returned once a year for three years. Gradually she stopped taking her medications, and her body returned to normal (though her eyes still had the popped-out appearance characteristic of Graves' disease).

The chakra system provides a practitioner with the most comprehensive holistic method for diagnosing illness. It gives information about the body (through the lower chakras), mind (through the third and sixth chakras), emotions (through the lower and middle chakras), and spirit (through the higher chakras). In Annette's case, we began with a physical ailment. Though she gave me a brief personal history, it wasn't until I felt the energy at her hips (her parents), her third chakra (center of power), and her throat chakra (center of communication) that she and I both understood the underlying cause of her illness. In Part 2, I will explain how to feel the energy at the chakras.

Annette's relationship with her mother led to a repression of energy at her throat chakra, causing a blockage that contributed to the thyroid disease. Once Annette was able to use the vibratory vehicle of her voice to express her suppressed rage, the flow of energy at her throat was released, and the T cells were jump-started so they could begin working properly.

Most medical doctors do not look for the underlying emotional cause of a physical disease. Even if Annette had been referred to a psychotherapist, it would have taken many months of talk therapy to sort out the problem, and even then, unless she was encouraged to scream, her thyroid glands would probably have remained dormant.

The goal of Vibrational Healing, as I see it, is to reach a perfect harmony of all seven chakras, in which the lower chakras of the physical body are open and balanced, the middle chakras of the emotions and personal power are open and balanced; and the higher chakras of intuition and spirituality are open and balanced, with no single chakra in control—except at appropriate times. Then the energies can move up and down the spine freely and the individual can be energetic, vitally alive, in touch with his emotions, and at peace.

In Annette's case, her hips gave information that helped me understand the origins of her disease. Her throat chakra began closing down when her spirit was broken as a small child. Her low self-esteem resulted from feeling that no one cared about her and being unable to express herself. Once she had permission to scream and release her pent-up feelings, she reclaimed her spirit and strengthened the energy at her throat chakra, which stimulated her T cells and drove out the disease.

## The Vibrational Healer

Machines have been developed that will give you a complete analysis of the colors that are missing in your energy field and the sounds that are lacking in your voice and body. These machines will bombard you with colored lights and sounds that are perfect for your body, and you will go away feeling better. Right?

Not necessarily. Some of these inventions are wonderful and can certainly contribute to your sense of well-being. But having a caring, compassionate practitioner is an essential part of healing. When you choose a Vibrational Healer, you must feel comfortable with that person. He or she should feel centered and balanced to you.

An understanding healer will be willing to meet with you on the phone or in person *before* you commit to a session. You should feel that you can talk about anything without being judged. If all of these qualifications are met, half the healing is already accomplished.

Russians Semyon and Valentina Kirlian developed a technique known as Kirlian photography that makes use of high-voltage spark discharges to provide a picture of the energy fields, which are often photographs taken from the thumbs of individuals being tested. Researchers found that when healers were at rest the corona of light around their thumbs were large and bright, whereas the patients had smaller coronas. During and after a healing, the auras of the healers actually decreased, while the auras of the patients increased sharply. This seems to indicate that there is a transfer of energy from the healer to the patient.[15]

You simply cannot do this work until your own chakras are reasonably cleansed, balanced, and aligned. The training for becoming a practitioner of this art is primarily Physician Heal Thyself. It is truly a journey of the soul.

It is essential for a practitioner to be willing to cancel a healing session if he or she is ill or "having a bad day." This is part of being human.

## History, Locations, and Numbers of Chakras

Various chakra systems exist, with different numbers, colors, and locations of chakras. Historically, there are various schools of thought about the locations of the chakras. Yet the basic four or five chakras are consistently placed in the same locations by all sources. The other chakras are found above, below, or between these basic chakras. Less powerful energy centers called lotuses or minor or extra chakras can be found at the feet, hands, knees, elbows, hips, shoulders, ears, and other places.

The use of the Sanskrit word, *chakra*, to describe spinning wheels of energy on or around the body first appeared in the ancient Hindu Upanishads around 200 B.C.E. The Brahma-Upanishad describes the four *purushas* (places occupied by the soul) at the navel, heart, throat, and head.

Tibetan Buddhism (Vajrayana Buddhism) acknowledges the same four centers as the Hindus, with the head center associated with the body, the throat center related to the dream state, and the heart center related to deep meditation. Other Tibetan systems mention five, seven, or even ten chakras. A painting from eighteenth-century Nepal, in south-central Asia, shows seven chakras, with the seventh clearly above the head.[16]

The Rosicrucian Order is believed to have been started in the 1400s by The Highly Illuminated Father C.R.C., a German by birth who at the age of sixteen traveled to Damascus in Syria when it was capital of the Islamic empire. There he was initiated into the secrets of Arabian adepts, including how to communicate with the elementals (nature spirits). When he returned to Europe, he translated a book called *M* that he brought back from his travels. But after being ridiculed, he gathered a secret society of eight followers who agreed to transcribe the teachings but to remain unknown to the world.[17]

The concept of energy centers was first brought to Western literature in the *Theosophia Practica* by the German Bavarian mystic Johann Georg Gichtel (1638–1710). Gichtel was a student of Jacob Boehme, who was probably a Rosicrucian. Gichtel, who had the gift of clairvoyance, saw the seven force centers through inner sight. He correlated them with the sun and the planets, placing the sun at the heart center. He founded a mystical Christian movement. In 1670 he was banished from Bavaria and took refuge in Holland.[18]

Between 600 and 800, the Roman Empire gave way to the Catholic Church, and Christianity became the ruling power in Europe. When religion combined with government, an unholy

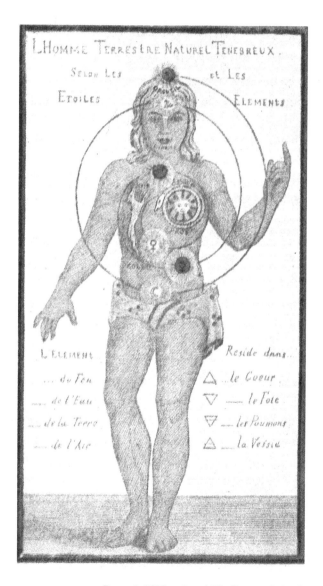

alliance was formed, and it became dangerous to use any form of healing not condoned by the church. People were no longer at liberty to choose their own religious or spiritual practices. Anything that interfered with the effectiveness of the church was considered an offense against God.

The fact that Gichtel was banished from his home in Bavaria and had to flee to Holland in 1670, and that a secret society formed in Europe during the Middle Ages is not surprising, given that the inquisition and the torture and burnings of so-called witches stretched from the fourteenth to the seventeenth centuries in Germany, Italy, Spain, France, and then in England and New England. This era of repression had deep repercussions in the areas of healing, as well as science and philosophy.

According to neuroscientist Candace Pert, the old idea of the mind being distinct from the body began with philosopher René Descartes (1596–1650). The mind/body separation "just goes back to a turf deal that Descartes made with the Roman Catholic Church. He got to study science, as we know it, and left the soul, the mind, the emotions, and consciousness to the realm of the church."[19]

Before the inquisition, women who were midwives and herbalists were the primary healers. Their services were available to poor and rich alike. These women were often great lovers of nature, gathering in small groups, to observe seasonal rituals that honored the power of the moon and the changes of the seasons. That was their religion.

The church considered these women heretics. Their power to heal was considered evidence that they were witches in league with the devil. All forms of healing used by these women were believed to be witchcraft, and it became the duty of monks in service to the pope to encourage villagers to reveal the presence of these so-called heretics so they could be punished and their souls could be saved. Some writers have estimated the total number killed to have been in the millions, though documented cases indicate 14,000 to 23,000.[20, 21]

While so-called witches were being tortured and burned, a new male medical profession was created and funded by the royalty, and universities were set up that excluded women. University-trained male doctors worked hand-in-hand with the church, calling in priests to aid and advise them, and refusing to treat patients who would not take confession.

The doctors of medieval times studied Socrates, Aristotle, and Christian theology, along with the works of the ancient Roman physician Galen, who wrote about "complexions" and "temperaments." Leeches were used for bleeding, along with certain foods, incantations, and rituals. Experimentation was not practiced, and there was no practicum and no apprenticeship. Surgery was performed by barbers, and dissection was virtually unheard of.

Towns and cities were filthy, and knowledge of hygiene was nonexistent. The Black Death killed one-third of England's population between 1340 and 1348. The cause of the Black Death according to Guy de Chauliac, a French doctor, was the convergence of three great planets, Saturn, Jupiter, and Mars, which was considered a clear sign of wonderful, terrible, or violent events.

Medieval peasants were taught by the church that illness could be a punishment from God for sinful behavior. Physicians charged well for their services, and only the rich could afford them. One of the most famous physicians was John Arderne who wrote "The Art of Medicine" and treated royalty. His cure for kidney stones was a hot plaster smeared with honey and pigeon dung.[22]

In 1875 in New York City, Madame Blavatsky (1831–1891) founded the Theosophical Society. The Theosophists believe in the presence of life and consciousness in all matter, the ability of thought to affect the reality we live in, and a concern for the welfare of others. Theosophists make use of meditation, and often support animal protection, ecology, and the rights of women and minorities.

Madame Blavatsky encouraged the study of Western mystical traditions such as gnosticism, the kabbalah, Freemasonry, and Rosicrucianism, as well as Buddhism. In 1878 she traveled to India. In 1884 she was defamed by the Society for Psychical Research (since repudiated by the Society) and moved to London. Later advocates of Theosophy include Annie Besant, Rudolf Steiner, and C. W. Leadbeater.

The Theosophical Society published Leadbeater's classic book, *The Chakras*, in 1927. His book included colored drawings of the seven chakras as Leadbeater saw them clairvoyantly. The swirls of colors in his drawings roughly follow the rainbow, with red hues at the first chakra, orange at the second, and so forth.

Sir John Woodroffe traveled from England to India, and when he returned, in 1928, he brought the Hindu interpretations of the chakras to the west by translating from Sanskrit two classic works on Laya-Yoga, the *Sat-Cakra-Nirupana* (1577) and *Paduka-Pancaka* (c. tenth century C.E.) in a book called *The Serpent Power*, published under the pen name of Arthur Avalon. His interpretations of the seven chakras and their locations concurred with those described by Leadbeater, and they became the model for the Theosophists. The Theosophists also ushered in the concept that the chakras are energy vortexes that have an independent objective existence associated with particular endocrine glands and nerve plexuses as well as specific vertebrae.

In his comprehensive study of the chakras, M. Alan Kazlev makes a distinction between those described by the Hindus, Buddhists, and Tibetans, which he calls Primary Chakras, and the Secondary Chakras described by the Theosophists and subsequent New Age proponents. Kazlev points out that in the Indian and Tibetan teachings, the yogi creates the chakras as part of his mental exercise, as a kind of visualization. Chakras are considered inactive until awakened through yoga. As the adept moves up through the chakras, the lower chakras close down as one attains full awareness at the higher chakras. On the other hand, what he calls the New Age or Secondary Chakras makes use of the rainbow system, in which the optimum goal is to be open at *all* the chakras.[23]

In *The Chakras*, Leadbeater also describes seven chakras in similar positions to those described by Woodroffe. He and other Theosophists agreed on the following names, vertebral locations, and nerve plexuses for these chakras:

First (coccygeal) at the fourth sacral—coccygeal plexus
Second (spleen) 20 at the first lumbar—splenic plexus[24]
Third (navel) at the eighth thoracic—solar plexus

Fourth (heart) at the eighth cervical—cardiac plexus

Fifth (throat) at the third cervical—pharyngeal plexus

Sixth (brow) at the first cervical—carotid plexus

Seventh (crown)—not related to the vertebrae or the plexuses[25]

In his exhaustive *Layayoga—an Advanced Method of Concentration* Shyam Sundar Goswami (1891–1978) describes the Shakta Theory of Chakras. The founder of the Goswami Institute of Yoga in Sweden, the first Indian institution of its kind in that country, he uses the same seven chakras found in *The Serpent Power*, adding six minor chakras, for a total of thirteen. He describes two chakras at the heart. I wonder if one might be the thymus gland, located several inches above the heart? He places another at the roof of the mouth. This is an important point in Chinese medicine, where the Yin Conception Vessel and the Yang Governing Vessel meet.

Goswami places two chakras at the forehead. This makes sense, since some sources show the third eye between the eyebrows and others show it at the center of the forehead. Finally he has three chakras at the crown. He places the Nirvana Chakra at the top of the head, the Guru Chakra above the head, and the Sahasrara Chakra also above the head. Most other systems place the Sahasrara Chakra at the very top of the head.[26]

Sri Aurobindo (1872–1950), a philosopher, yogi, and teacher in India, was educated in England and influenced by the Theosophists. He returned to India and developed Integral Yoga, the yoga of the whole being. He described the seven chakras found in *Serpent Power* and related each one to an aspect of psychology. For example, he indicated that the first chakra governed "the physical down to the subconscient [subconsious]".[27]

Other sources describe chakras above the crown. Some call these the transpersonal chakras, and they are often related to the higher vibrations of light and sound. Yet another system has twenty chakras, including two below the base chakra that link to the earth and others above the head that link to the cosmos.

The Hesychastic tradition in the Eastern Orthodox or Byzantine Church combines breathing techniques with prayer in a form of contemplative Christianity. They practice concentrating on four different parts of the body: 1) the eyebrows (related to thought); 2) the base of the neck (related to conversation); 3) the upper and median region of the chest (related to thought and emotions); and 4) a little below the left breast (the physical site of perfect attention).[28]

Chakras can be found in the teachings of Jesus Christ. When Joseph and Mary were escaping from Herod they fled to Egypt. It is not unlikely, as some sources claim, that Jesus was educated in the Far East. In Luke 11:34 Jesus said, "The light of the body is the eye: therefore when thine eye is single, thy whole body also is full of light; but when thine eye is evil, thy body also is full of darkness." The third eye is the sixth chakra, which is known as the Christ Consciousness Center.

In Olga Kharitidi's book, *Entering the Circle: Ancient Secrets of Siberian Wisdom Discovered by a Russian Psychiatrist*, she describes her initiation with a Siberian shaman. Kharitidi claims that many original religions were influenced by an ancient civilization that flourished in Siberia when the weather was warm, before a sudden change in climate. These include people who later gave birth to Zoroastranism in Iran, the Vedic tradition of India, Tantric Buddhism in Tibet, and the Celts in England.[29] It is interesting that some Hopi Indians trace their migration to North America back to ancient times when they came across the Siberian Straits, when the continents were connected.[30]

The Hopi Indians brought the knowledge of the chakras to the West long before the Theosophists. In Frank Waters's *Book of the Hopi*, Oswald White Bear Fredericks, himself a Hopi, interviewed 26 Hopi spokesmen. The Hopi speak about four worlds.

The first world came to an end when few of the original people lived by the laws of Creation. "More and more they used the vibratory centers of their bodies solely for earthly purposes." In a story that sounds remarkably like the Wise Men of the East following the star to the Christ Child, the few who continued in the old ways were told, "You go to a certain place. Your *kopavi* [vibratory center at the top of the head at the seventh chakra] will lead you. This inner wisdom will give you the sight to see a certain cloud which you will follow by day, and a certain star, which you will follow by night." When all the people arrived from different places, the chosen ones went down and lived in the ant *kiva* (a round underground room) while the rest of the world was destroyed.

The Hopi describe five vibratory centers. In remarkable agreement with the Hindus, they begin on top, with the soft spot, *kopavi*, the "open door" through which a person receives life and communicates with his Creator. It remains closed until his death, "opening then for his life to depart as it had come."

The second center corresponds to the brain. The third center, at the throat, is a center of communication in both cultures. The fourth center is at the heart. The Hopi say, "In his heart man felt the good of life, its sincere purpose. He was of One Heart. But there were those who permitted evil feelings to enter. They were said to be of Two Hearts."

The fifth and last Hopi chakra is located at the navel. In other systems this chakra is described as being directly at the navel, or an inch or two above the navel. It is associated with personal and worldly power. For the Hopi "it was the throne in man of the Creator himself. From it he directed all the functions of man."[31]

In *Serpent Power*, Sir John Woodroffe mentions that some of the Sufi fraternities use the kundalini method (see Glossary) as a means to realization, and he also draws correlations with the Mayan scripture, the Popul Vuh, as containing references to the kundalini and the chakras.[32]

In her book *Sacred Contracts*, Caroline Myss, a medical intuitive, describes the archetypes that she perceives as the organizing principle for the life contracts that we assume prior to birth. She perceives these universal archetypes as coming through a location above each person's head that she describes as the eighth chakra.[33]

I experience a strong similarity between the first and second chakras, and also between the sixth and seventh chakras. So it does not surprise me to find systems that describe only five chakras.

Some systems talk about a chakra at the navel, and others talk about a chakra above the navel. I feel that the one at the navel is the same as the third chakra above the navel.

The heart chakra stands alone. It does not merge with the others. Virtually every system agrees that there is a chakra at the center of the chest. There is even agreement about the sound *ah* at that chakra. Most systems agree on the colors green and/or pink for the heart chakra.

All systems concur that there is a chakra at the third eye. Some place it between the eyebrows; some at the center of the forehead; some a little higher. When a crown chakra is identified, some say it is at the top of the head, and others say it is above the top of the head.

Barbara Ann Brennan began seeing energy fields as a child. Later she became a research scientist for NASA at the Goddard Space Flight Center. In 1972 she began to work with the human energy field, and in 1987 she wrote *Hands of Light*.

According to Brennan, a different energy can be felt at the back of each of the chakras. One can visualize a beam of energy shooting through the body from the front and emerging out the back. Brennan describes these energy centers as bulging out in front and back of the body at the chakra centers, with the crown and base chakras being opposite ends of one long double megaphone.[34]

Some sources, however, say that the back of the sixth chakra is at the base of the skull, at the medulla oblongata.

Don't let these discrepancies bother you. Choose a system that works for you, use it repeatedly and then be willing to deviate from it, just as you might learn to play scales on a musical instrument and then learn to improvise. You might even play overtones—notes that aren't actually on the keyboard or in the musical notation. In fact, there are many different scales: chromatic, diatonic, and pentatonic. That doesn't mean only one scale is right (though the others may sound peculiar to your ear, and may not resonate for you). There are different ways of perceiving reality and different systems for ordering the universe.

## Colors of the Chakras

Dr. Valerie Hunt worked with eight aura readers while recording chakra frequencies with her highly sensitive equipment. She writes:

Often aura readers reported. . . . red in the coccyx, orange in the abdomen, yellow in the solar plexus, green in the heart, blue in the throat, violet in the third eye, and white in the crown—although this was not always the case. . . .

Furthermore, the sensor readings from chakra locations corresponded directly with aura readers' descriptions of amount of energy, its color, and the dynamic quality. In addition, there seemed to be a close relationship between these measures and the emotional states, imagery, and interpersonal transactions of the subjects.[35]

It is difficult to assign colors to the chakras. They are not stable and constant like the red, amber, and green of traffic lights. Clairvoyants describe the chakras as shimmering, fluctuating, constantly changing. Some say they follow the colors of the rainbow. But the Indians and Tibetans used red, white, blue, smoke, and so forth.

Let's look at some descriptions of the chakras, as seen by those who have the gift of clairvoyance. C.W. Leadbeater referred to "The brilliant colouring and the rapid and incessant movement of the chakras. . . . When quite undeveloped they appear as small circles about two inches in diameter, glowing dully in the ordinary man, but when awakened and vivified they are seen as blazing, coruscating whirlpools, much increased in size, and resembling miniature suns."

To see these emanations, says Leadbeater, is "to make oneself sensitive to vibrations more rapid than those to which our physical senses are normally trained to respond." He describes "a series of wheel-like vortices which exist in the surface of the etheric double of man. All these wheels are perpetually rotating, and into the hub or open mouth of each a force from the higher world is always flowing. . . The primary force itself, having entered the vortex, radiates from it again at right angles, but in straight lines, as though the hub of the vortex were the hub of a wheel."[36]

Most sources agree that the colors change as the emotions change, and at any given moment they can be clouded over, brilliant, or obscured. For the sake of simplicity, I speak of seven colors, but in truth, there are a wide variety of colors that each chakra can display.

Dr. Hunt said, "I use red, orange and amber [together] because the spectrum is so close that you really can't separate them. . . . It modulates." She also spoke about a merging of blue, mauve, and violet in the higher chakras.[37]

There are many instances of people who have seen the chakras, even when they had no previous concept of their existence. One doctor who inadvertently discovered his own clairvoyance was W. Brugh Joy, a heart and lung specialist from the University of Southern California. "I was examining a healthy male in his early twenties," he explained. "As my hand passed over the solar plexus area, the pit of the stomach, I sensed something that felt like a warm cloud. It seemed to radiate out three to four feet from the body, perpendicular to the surface, and to be shaped like a cylinder about four inches in diameter."[38] Apparently he was feeling the third chakra.

In the 1960s, neurologist and psychiatrist Shafica Karagulla found that she could see the human energy field. She began interviewing other medical professionals including famous surgeons, Cornell University professors of medicine, heads of departments in large hospitals, and Mayo Clinic physicians. Karagulla met doctor after doctor who had this ability. As she explains in her book, *Breakthrough to Creativity*, they would describe an "energy field" or a "moving web of frequency" around and interpenetrating the body. One described "vortices of energy at certain points along the spine, connected with or influencing the endocrine system."[39]

## The Rainbow System

The rainbow system that I use consists of seven chakras, from the tailbone to the top of the head. They follow the colors of the rainbow: red, orange, yellow, green, blue, indigo (or violet), and violet (or white). When a person has achieved enlightenment, or is fully integrated and balanced, all the chakras are fully open, and the color of the aura is white (the combination of all colors). This is depicted by Christian artists as a halo around the heads of saints and holy figures.

Primarily through the higher chakras we receive energy from the light body and from All That Is. Primarily through the lower chakras we receive energy from the earth. Primarily through the middle chakras we exchange energies with other people and animals.

Here are the locations and colors of the seven major chakras in the Rainbow System:

First—Red (at the tailbone)
Second—Orange (below the navel)
Third—Yellow (above the navel, at the solar plexus)
Fourth—Green & Pink (at the heart)
Fifth—Blue (at the throat)
Sixth—Indigo or Violet (at the center of the forehead)
Seventh—Violet or White (at the crown of the head)

The lower two chakras (first and second) open when in the presence of nature or through yoga and other pleasurable forms of exercise and lovemaking. The third chakra opens through a sense of personal fulfillment. The fourth chakra opens when you can give and receive unconditional love. The fifth chakra opens during communication. The sixth chakra opens when you enter into communion with the psychic and spiritual realms. The seventh chakra opens with deep meditation and when you feel connected with Spirit.

The relative openness of the chakras determines your ability to receive and generate energy. Each of the chakras is governed by a particular vibration, which may be interpreted as a color or sound. The aura is a reflection of the combined frequencies of the chakras and is generally predominated by one or two colors, which flow from the strongest chakras. When all the chakras are open, and all the colors/vibrations run together in relatively equal proportions, the aura becomes white.

## Science of the Chakras

The chakras exist in the energy field, which is nonphysical; it is constantly fluctuating, vibrating, ephemeral. It interacts with people and with the environment *and* with the observer. So nothing absolutely objective and conclusive can be said about the chakras. Yet there are scientists who are finding evidence for their existence.

In the early 1970s, Dr. Valerie Hunt openly encouraged her physiology students at the University of California, Los Angeles to explore the parameters of consciousness, including the parapsychological. She was taken aback by the overwhelming interest her students showed in these areas. Then a graduate student asked Dr. Hunt to run tests to help her understand what happened when she went into an "altered state" while dancing.

"At that time," explains Hunt in her book, *Infinite Mind*, "an altered state seemed unreal to me, for there were no guidelines as to how to record consciousness, and no agreement even as to what it was."

Instead of stating—as most scientists did in the 1970s—that there was no such thing as an "altered state" (a highly unscientific attitude), she gave it a lot of thought. A few weeks later she came up with a plan.

> Possibly the neurological level of muscle stimulation held a clue to consciousness levels. Timidly, I placed the electromyographic (EMG) recording electrodes on her lower arm, her upper arm, and her back muscles, each area primarily stimulated by a different level of the spinal cord and brain. Intuitively, in a playful mood, I placed one electrode on top of her head, although I knew nothing about chakras. . . .
>
> In five minutes the recordings remarkably changed. The muscular signal from her lower arm stopped. The baseline activity

characteristic of all living tissue was absent on the scopes. Next, the upper arm recording dropped out. The engineer believed there was no equipment failure, although there was no ordinary energy in the arms. Soon she sat down in a "tailor position". . . . Next, electromagnetic energy poured from the top of her head with intensity beyond what our equipment could handle. This state lasted for seven minutes, followed by a reverse sequence of reactivating the spine, upper arm, and lower arm muscles. . . . I was at a total loss to explain, but I could not forget these happenings.[40]

Later Hunt received a grant to study the energetic effects of Rolfing, a form of deep tissue bodywork originated in the 1940s by Ida P. Rolf. Dr. Hunt knew that ordinary equipment was incapable of detecting the minute signals of the energy field, so she approached an engineer who developed highly sensitive telemetry systems for NASA to record astronauts' heart and muscle activity while in space. She asked him to build the unique instrument that she used for her experiments.

Telemetry is a radio broadcasting system that intercepts and projects the body's electrical activity. Surface sensors pick up the body's electrical signals by FM radio frequency carrier via a miniature, battery-operated radio transmitter and amplifier attached to the subject by a belt. The airborne signal is then picked up by a radio receiver and recorded on tape or disk. Dr. Hunt's data were analyzed by data analysis procedures such as Wave Shape Analysis, Fourier Frequency Analysis, and Frequency Spectrogram, all of which produced consistent results.

The telemetry instrument enabled Dr. Hunt to record regular, high-frequency electrical oscillations coming from the chakras that had never been previously recorded or reported in the scientific literature. Traditionally scientists thought of biological energy as that which takes place in the activity of the brain waves, or in the shortening and lengthening of the muscles, including the beating of the heart. Brain wave activity is measured by an electroencephalogram (EEG, between zero and 200 cycles per second (cps). The heart's electrical activity is recorded by an electrocardiogram (EKG), which creates a larger and faster wave at about 225 cps. The electrical current produced when a muscle shortens can be recorded by an electromyogram (EMG), with a wider range, from zero to 250 cps.

Conventional recordings are taken by inserting needle sensors or probes into a nerve or muscle, which gives a reading only for the very local electricity. Dr. Hunt attached the electrodes to the surface of the skin where there was a larger signal. She amplified the baseline on the oscilloscope and filtered the data to remove the brain, heart, and muscle frequencies. She discovered a void of electrical activity between about 250 and 500 cps, and then she discovered a continuous activity from 500 to 20,000 cps (the highest capacity of the instrument at the time.)[41]

In one of Hunt's studies, Emilie, who was a healer, worked with a congenitally brain-disturbed young man who had been evaluated as having abnormal brain waves. An aura reader, Rosalyn Bruyere (who has since become quite famous—the movie *Resurrection* is based on her life) was brought in to read the colors and describe activity that she observed in the energy field.

Dr. Hunt applied surface sensors on the young man's skin over the areas that were alleged to relate to the chakras. A data-tape was set up to record Emilie's shamanic chanting, Rosalyn's descriptions, and Dr. Hunt's narration of the healer's movements. For three hours, "Emilie performed esoteric movements around his body and shouted into his kneecaps. She shook rattles and bells, and waved crystals around his body, but she never touched him."

At the end of three hours the young man's brain waves had stabilized into a normal pattern. When all the data were analyzed, there was only one firm relationship.

> There was a very close correlation between what the aura reader said and the gross happenings in the electrical activity of the man's auric field. For example, when Rosalyn reported energy entering his arm, the amplitude of the recordings increased. She described that energy had entered his feet and progressed up his legs, "shooting the Kundalini" and "getting balled up in the heart chakra."

These unscientific descriptions were nonetheless synchronized with the electronic data showing sudden energy flowing up both legs with an increased amplitude in the lower abdomen, or Kundalini, and stopping in the heart chakra. The chart showed a two-fold increase in the amplitude of contraction with no change in the rate.

Rosalyn's next description convinced me that some unknown energy was flowing when she described that Emilie had released the energy from the heart which spurted out the crown chakra on top of the head in bursts of white light. The spurts were in sync with the sudden energy bursts which came from the crown electrodes, and the frequencies of these data were the highest recorded during that session.

The sensor readings from the chakras corresponded directly with the aura reader's descriptions, including amount of energy, color, and dynamic quality.[42]

In another study, Dr. Hiroshi Motoyama of Japan speculated that since the chakras are believed to be transformers that bring energy into the body and transmit energy out of the body, it seemed reasonable to assume that highly aware persons could consciously project energy out of their chakras. While Motoyama had no way of measuring the primary subtle energy of the chakras, he hoped to measure secondary energy, such as electrostatic fields.

Choosing subjects who were advanced meditators and those with previous psychic experiences, he placed electrodes in front of chakras that the subjects claimed had been awakened. By measuring the amplitude and frequency of the electrical field at the presumed chakras, Motoyama found that the level of energy at these locations was significantly greater than the recordings made at the corresponding areas of the control subjects.

Motoyama also monitored the energy that the advanced meditators claimed to be able to project through their chakras. He documented significant electrical field disturbances emanating from the activated chakras. These results were repeated by Motoyama over a number of years and later by Itzhak Bentov, author of *Stalking the Wild Pendulum,* who successfully used similar equipment to duplicate Motoyama's findings.[43]

## Different Realities

An old Cherokee was teaching his grandchildren about life. He said to them, "A fight is going on inside me. It is a terrible fight, and it is between two wolves. One wolf represents fear, anger, envy, sorrow, regret, greed, arrogance, self-pity, guilt, resentment, inferiority, lies, false pride, superiority, and ego.

"The other stands for joy, peace, love, hope, sharing, serenity, humility, kindness, benevolence, friendship, empathy, generosity, truth, compassion, and faith.

"This same fight is going on inside you, and inside every other person, too."

They thought about it for a minute, and then one child asked his grandfather, "Which wolf will win?"

The old man simply replied, "The one you feed."

It amazes me that different cultures independently had similar concepts about something that is invisible. However, I am not particularly surprised that there is not perfect agreement about how many chakras there are or what their colors are. If you can find a system that works for you, it doesn't have to be consistent with other systems. Just having a clear intent seems more important than having agreement about exactly what it looks like. Some physicists believe that the strength of the observer's intention will influence the form that a subatomic particle will assume.

In the 1930s, eminent physicist Wolfgang Pauli (who coauthored a book with psychologist Carl Jung), proposed the existence of a massless particle called a neutrino to solve a problem about radioactivity. In 1980 evidence was found in the Soviet Union that the neutrino possessed a small but measurable mass. Labs in the United States could not duplicate these findings for many years. This caused some experts to speculate about whether it might be possible for different properties displayed by neutrinos to be due, in part, to the changing expectations and cultural biases of the physicist who searched for them.[44]

This might explain why in the United States the much-touted ability of aspirin to decrease the risk of heart attack is completely ineffective in England, where a six-year study of 5,139 British doctors showed no evidence that aspirin reduced that risk.[45]

Barbara Brennan, the author of *Hands of Light*, has her own distinct concept of what the chakras look like, where they are located, and how they function. She presents that concept to her students, and they believe it, work with it, and make it so.

I have my own clear sense of what the chakras are—where they are, what they do, what their colors are, what their functions are, and how they work. My system works well for me and my students, and I use it on my clients with great benefit. So I will share this system that I have used for nineteen years, feeling the spin of energy at the chakras of thousands of people.

My belief is that, if you resonate with a system, it will probably work for you. That is the most important criterion because, in the world of energy, your mental expectations are likely to have a profound effect upon the reality that you experience. There is nothing wrong with that. In fact, it is perfectly scientific.

Human beings are organizers of reality, and your reality will conform to the organizing principles that you impose upon it. When you truly grasp this concept, you will understand how you create your own reality and how you can transform the reality that you create.

## Opening and Closing of the Chakras

As you go through life, you respond to various events by opening up or closing down physically, emotionally, and/or spiritually. Theoretically, a person who is fully enlightened is totally open at all the chakras and is not susceptible to these kinds of fluctuations.

When your spirit enters your body, which usually occurs when you are still in the womb, all your chakras are open. Newborn babies who are truly wanted and who experience natural childbirth tend to be unarmored, energetic, and completely in tune with All That Is. But even in the womb and during birth, many babies experience a closing off of the energy centers. Rejection can be experienced long before birth.

The chakras tend to close down from the top downward. In my work with hypnotherapy, I observed that most people close down their top three chakras by the time they are three years old, as a reaction to the disbelief of their parents and society (in nature spirits, spirit friends, angels, past life experiences, and Spirit). During the teenage years, the heart chakra often closes down or becomes imbalanced because of pain and rejection from parents, peers, and lovers. The third chakra often closes down or becomes imbalanced when parents and society force teens into molds that do not fit. By the time they enter adulthood, many people close down all but the first two or three chakras. The relative closure of a chakra does not ordinarily occur because of a single event; it is the response to the frequent repetition of similar events.

After high school, there is less pressure to conform. Some people begin to reverse the process and start opening their chakras. Usually the third chakra opens first. Eventually all the chakras may open in succession, going upward. But that isn't always the case. For example, I've worked with people who were spiritually developed in past lives, but in their current lifetime came from difficult family situations and had little sense of self-worth. These people did not need to work on their higher chakras to become whole; they needed to work on their lower chakras. They needed to have a full experience of living in their bodies, feeling their sexuality, and discovering the joy and beauty of nature.

Please note: When I speak about the chakras "closing down," I do not mean that they are totally closed, but that they are at least 50 percent closed.

## Author's Experience with the Chakras

My main teacher for the chakras is a Spirit Guide named Dr. Laing. He came to me when I was in my late twenties. The reason

Dr. Laing chose to work with me is a story worth telling. His only beloved daughter discovered the Theosophists (see Glossary) and was exuberant about how the colorful whorls of energy called chakras could revolutionize the art of healing.

Dr. Laing listened patiently to his offspring when she returned home late at night from their meetings, but he was convinced that the ideas of the Theosophists were childish and irrelevant. Finally he would lose patience, begging her to ignore those "charlatans."

When his daughter was twenty-one, she died in an accident. Laing mourned her for the rest of his life. When he died, he was amazed to find himself in his astral body, from which he could see the colored whorls of energy around human bodies. He discovered that when the colors were faded or cloudy or blotchy he could detect the beginnings of illness before symptoms occurred in the physical body. He was so deeply moved by this revelation that he resolved to become his daughter's Spirit Guide in one of her future lifetimes, so that by working on both planes they could bring this consciousness to humanity. Dr Laing is not to be confused with Dr. William Lang, a guide who worked through Theosophist George Chapman in England. Nor should he be confused with R. D. Laing, a contemporary psychologist.

Laing approached me in 1979. He would show up (usually during long trips, when I was driving alone) and lecture me for an hour at a time. Eventually he told me that I had been his daughter. The main focus of his lectures turned to the use of color for healing and inner growth. He organized these lectures around the chakras, beginning with the first and moving upward. At that time I knew little about the chakras, and had not even heard of color healing

Balancing the chakras through the use of color was an entirely new concept in the United States. Laing was trying to teach me and now I was the skeptical one. Feeling distrustful, I searched through books, unable to find anything about chakras or color healing. Finally, in a metaphysical bookstore, I found *The Serpent Power* by Sir John Woodroffe, *The Chakras*, by C. W. Leadbeater, and *Colour Healing* by Mary Anderson—all from England.

(Today you can go into the search engine on Google.com on the Internet and do a search for "chakra" and get 805,000 entries. In January 2005, Amazon.com lists 391 books on the chakras and 366 on color healing.)

I was amazed that the information in Mary Anderson's book dovetailed perfectly with Laing's. His descriptions of the personality types that correspond with each chakra went a step beyond her book. Later I found that Christopher Hills described the chakra personality types in *Nuclear Evolution*, published in the 1970s. His information is similar to that which I received from Dr. Laing in 1979. In 1997 Ambika Wauters wrote about *Chakras and their Archetypes*, and her perceptions are also similar to Laing's.

Laing was born before the turn of the century in India. His father was a British doctor, and both parents were mystics. Laing returned to England where he worked as a conventional doctor during the late nineteenth and early twentieth centuries.

After Laing introduced me to the chakras, I discovered Katrina Raphaell's book, *Crystal Enlightenment*, which opened up a whole new understanding of the crystals. Then Laing began channeling specific information about different kinds of clear quartz crystals, and I began to receive information directly from the stones. I found myself placing stones on my clients. I was astonished by how powerful they were. Whether I was doing a past life regression or hypnosis or clearing the chakras or working on emotional release, everything was easier and went faster when I used the stones.

In 1986, while I was teaching a workshop on Color, Sound, Crystals, and the Chakras at Paul Pitchford's Holistic Healing Retreat in Idaho, I was approached by an opera singer from New York. She offered to demonstrate a method she learned for feeling the energy of the chakras. I lay down on the massage table and she held a long thin crystal a few inches above my body, aiming the point at each chakra while moving it in a circular direction.

As she felt the energy at each center, she uttered strange, unfamiliar sounds that had an uncanny emotional depth, as if she were able to feel my emotions and give voice to them. The sounds of the lower chakras were deep and gutteral, and as she moved up toward my head, the sounds became high and otherworldly.

"Your energy is balanced," she remarked. "You have your feet on the ground and your head in the heavens. That's unusual."

When she reached my third eye, she made a piercing sound that entered my skull like a drill. Then she announced with authority, "You have done this work in a past life, and you will do it again." I knew she was referring to the work she was doing on me.

I experienced a dull pain at my third eye for several days after the session and then, without further instruction, I obtained a long thin crystal and began using it to "feel" the energy at the chakras. The work came naturally to me.

Over the next year, I developed my own system of Chakra Diagnosis and a unique method of Vibrational Alignment™ for balancing the chakras. Over the years I correlated the use of crystals, sound, and aromatherapy with the chakras. These are the primary methods that I use and teach today.

## Chakra Diagnosis

I will now describe how to do chakra diagnosis and in the next section, Vibrational Alightment™, but please do not use these techniques professionally until you have been certified through the Vibrational Healing Program (see Resources). *Do not attempt to use these techniques unless you have a strong background in counseling and listening to your inner voice. CAUTION: Vibrational Healing is designed to facilitate a person's own self-healing. It is not intended to take the place of a doctor or a psychologist.*

Chakra diagnosis is a method of retrieving information about the body, mind, emotions, and spirit to form a coherent picture of the whole person. Psychologists, counselors, and energy healers find this information invaluable for understanding the inner journeys of their clients.

Clinical psychologist Ronald Wong Jue, former president of the Association for Transpersonal Psychology, uses a similar method of diagnosis that he calls Holographic Body Assessment.

"The body is a kind of microcosm, a universe unto itself reflecting all of the different factors that a person is dealing with and trying to integrate," he says. He lays his hands on a person's body and then tunes in to "movies" about the important issues in that person's life, including emotional scripts, core issues, and relationship patterns. He then uses this information to facilitate the therapeutic process. [46]

Chakra diagnosis is a similar method that does not involve touching the physical body. The Vibrational Healer holds a long thin crystal a couple inches above each chakra, moving it in a circular direction until she receives information in the form of sensations, visual images, or past-life pictures.

The practitioner can feel the degree to which each chakra is open or closed. People can be trained to do this, but individuals have different psychic skills: one person sees auras, another hears voices, and yet another feels energies. Feeling the energy of the chakras is a gift that comes easily to many, though some find they have stronger gifts in other areas. For example, I do not (as yet) see auras, but I am proficient at feeling the spin of the chakras.

If you want to feel the energy of the chakras, sit alongside your friend or client. If you are right-handed, sit with your right hand toward his feet and your left toward his head. Use your right hand to feel the feet, legs, and first five chakras. Use your left hand to feel the top two chakras. If you are left-handed, do the reverse. Your client may lie prone on a massage table, couch, or bed. If necessary, a light blanket may be used. You may offer a small pillow for his head and a larger pillow under his knees.

Hold a long, thin, single-terminated (single-pointed) clear quartz crystal a couple inches above each chakra. I use a crystal that is about six inches long and about ¾ inch in diameter. It can be formed naturally or shaped. You may prefer to use just your hand, but most people find that the crystal magnifies the energy.

Instead of a crystal, you may wish to use a pendulum (see Glossary). When a pendulum is suspended over each chakra, it may make a circular movement, and the size and strength of the spin will give an indication of the relative openness of the chakra. Do not be discouraged if you do not feel or see the energy clearly at first. This method is taught in my program only after four weeks of preparation.

Hold the crystal at its base with the termination pointing toward the chakra. Relax your hand as you move it in a counterclockwise circle a couple inches from the chakra. Wait until you feel caught up in the energy, as if you were stirring a pot of soup, feeling the thickness of the broth. In addition to feeling the size and speed of the energy, you may experience visual images, emotions, bodily sensations, sounds, tastes, or smells.

In my experience, the chakras spin in a clockwise direction, as electromagnetic energy does. When feeling the energy of the chakras, go counterclockwise at first, as if you were going against the tide to feel the pull of the tide. This also helps unwind negative energy. Begin at the feet (see below) and go through each chakra until you reach the crown. Then go clockwise from the crown, back down to the feet to restore the normal spin.

The left side relates to the client's feminine nature and tends to be influenced by his mother. The right side relates to his masculine nature and tends to be influenced by his father. As you feel the energy, think about the following:

Feet—Is he on his life path? Is he going forward in life?

Knees—How does he feel about responsibility?

Hips—How did his mother (left side) and father (right side) feel about him during the first three years of his life and prenatally (while he was in the womb)? How did they feel about being parents?

First chakra (at the tailbone)—Did he receive unconditional love and physical affection as a child? How strong is his will to survive? How grounded does he feel? How good is he at manifesting the objects of his desires? Is he comfortable in his body?

Second chakra (below the navel)—How does he feel about his sexuality? Is he comfortable socializing? How strong is his desire, not just sexual desire, but the desire for anything: friends, love, material possessions, God. Can he manifest what he needs and wants?

Third chakra (at the solar plexus, above the navel, or at the navel)—How does he feel about himself? Is he self-confident?

Does he know what his gift for the world is, and is he expressing it? Does his inner sun shine brightly? Is his digestion strong or weak? (All the digestive organs except the large intestines are located here.)

Fourth chakra (at the chest)—Does he have walls around his heart? How dense are they? Can he give and receive unconditional love and affection?

Fifth chakra (at the base of the throat)—Is he a good communicator? Does he speak well in public? Is he comfortable singing? Does his creativity flow easily?

Sixth chakra (at the center of the forehead)—Is he open to metaphysical insights? Is he in touch with his higher intuition?

Seventh chakra (at the top of the head)—Is he open to Spirit? Is he on a spiritual path that feels fulfilling to him?

A healthy open chakra is about the size of a person's open hand, with the diameter stretching from the tip of her thumb to the tip of her little finger. A large person with large hands would have proportionately larger chakras. But the energy emanating from and received by a smaller person would not necessarily be weaker, just as a small diamond is not diminished in radiance just because it is smaller than a larger quartz crystal.

When the energy at a given chakra is balanced and strong, the wheel of energy will move freely and easily without encountering obstructions. It may give off emanations and pulsations, or it may spiral upward, perpendicular to the table. The radiance emanating from an open chakra can stretch a great distance.

There are approximately seven stages of openness at each chakra. I will describe what I feel at each of the seven stages and how I interpret what I feel, going from the smallest to the largest amount of energy. Remember that this is a highly subjective experience.

Almost closed—You can barely find the spin of energy. It feels lifeless and weak. The circle is about the size of a dime. This chakra has just enough energy to keep the corresponding internal organs and endo-crine glands functioning. When a chakra is this weak, a person is highly susceptible to disease and may be dying.

Slightly open—The energy is slow and lethargic. The size of the circle is no larger than a quarter. This chakra is functioning at a minimal level. This person has low resistance to infection, and her will to live is not strong.

Less than half open—The spin of energy is sluggish and lacks enthusiasm. The size of the spin is no more than a silver dollar. This chakra is functional and the energy is adequate but weak.

More than half open—The energy spins a little slower than the pace of the heart. The size of the spin is about as large as the open palm of the person's hand. This is normal and healthy.

Average openness—The energy spins at the pace of the heart. The spin is about the size of the palm, plus the first digit of the fingers. This chakra feels energetic and in good health.

Wide open—The energy spins at the pace of the heart. The size of the spin is the size of the entire hand including the fingers. This chakra exudes radiant, dynamic, enthusiastic energy.

Extremely open—The energy spins at the pace of the heart. The diameter of the spin is that of two open hands. The energy is strong, and the circle is well formed and highly coherent. This person is exultant and basking in light.

Excessively open—This energy feels excessive. The spin exceeds the size of her open hand (including the fingers) yet lacks coherence, has an undefined shape, and feels weak and thin. It may be extremely fast or slow. It may feel like oil on water, spreading out aimlessly. This occurs when a person has "spread herself too thin." It is roughly comparable to the third stage of openness (less than half open).

There are other times when the spin is very large, up to two or three feet in diameter, but the substance of the energy feels weak. This occurs when a person "overextends himself" or "loves too much."

Usually the energy will be felt in a relatively flat plane, but sometimes it spirals upward from the body (when the person is lying down). This is usually a positive emanation, characteristic of the later stages of openness. But it can also occur when a person feels the need to escape from her body. For example, if an adolescent girl has spiraling energy at her second chakra, she may be leaving her body as a way of escaping sexual abuse.

When I first developed this technique, I noticed distinct correlations. For example, when I held the crystal at a person's left hip I received images and sensations related to his or her mother, and I often experienced that person as a baby or small child. After feeling the energy at the hips of about a hundred people, I concluded that the left hip holds the energy of the mother and the right hip holds the energy of the father—during the first three years of life and prenatally.

I was amazed by the complexity of information I received. It was like doing a psychic reading at each chakra. Sometimes I seemed to enter into the body and the psyche of a person's parents. I could talk for five or ten minutes about a person's mother: how she felt about being a mom, how she felt about this baby, whether she was happy or depressed or distracted, how she felt about herself, how she felt about her husband.

The information I received was usually extremely accurate, including fine details. For example, when I felt the energy at one woman's left hip, I felt a sense of enthusiastic, happy energy in half the circle while the other half felt depressed. When I asked if this made sense to her, the woman responded that her birth mother—who was good-natured and loved her very much—died when she was one year old. Then her father remarried. Her new mother suffered from deep depressions. The fact that this is possible implies that we carry the earliest imprint of our parents' emotional bodies with us throughout our lifetimes.

## Vibrational Alignment™

The Vibrational Alignment™ is a unique and powerful technique that I have developed over the past fifteen years. If you attempt to use this technique professionally do not call it by this name until you have been certified through the Vibrational Healing Program (see Resources). This process combines intuitive counseling and chakra diagnosis with a broad range of transpersonal healing modalities including the use of the vibratory tools. It brings the energy of the chakras into balance and brings the body into harmonious alignment with the earth and the heavens. In a future book, I will describe and explain the other modalities that I use and teach.

Begin a session by sitting and speaking with your client. You may serve tea. This is a relaxed time. Especially if this is someone new, you want to get to know each other, to establish trust and overcome anxiety. A client who is apprehensive will be in resistance, and you will have to work twice as hard to break through his armoring. Time spent relaxing will further every aspect of the work.

You may simply speak about the weather or his family, or simple non-threatening topics. Or your client may break down in tears and pour out his soul. It doesn't matter. He doesn't need to say anything at all, because the energy of the chakras will reveal everything.

When the client is relaxed, receptive, and trusting (in an alpha state or deeper), his energies will entrain to the energies of the vibratory tools and to your energies, so it is imperative for you to be relaxed and centered.

A Vibrational Healer will always deliver his own vibrations along with the stones, aromas and sounds. A Vibrational Healer is more like a midwife than a doctor: facilitating, sharing tools, providing a safe place to get in touch with and release pent-up feelings, giving unconditional love so the client feels empowered to do whatever she needs for her own healing.

It isn't necessary for a client to believe in Vibrational Healing. Healthy skepticism is fine. Why should she believe in what she has not experienced? But if she has actual resistance, there is no point in doing the work. This work requires full active participation on the part of the client. It is a partnership. You can act as a guide, a midwife. But the client needs to want to have the baby. For this reason I always ask individuals to make their own appointments. If a woman is pressuring her husband to see me, it is unlikely that we will have a productive session. Every treatment is like a jigsaw puzzle. All the pieces fit together and make perfect sense by the time you feel all the chakras from the feet to the top of the head. For example, a problem may show up in the feet that will almost certainly appear again at the hips or third chakra, because walking your path (the feet) is affected by how you feel about yourself and how you express your inner power (third chakra), and it is often influenced by your mother and/or your father in your early life (hips). A problem at the knees (responsibility) will also be affected by the hips and third chakra, for similiar reasons. The energy at the hips (your parents) can affect every other chakra, particularly the first (grounding), third (personal power), and fifth (confidence in communication). Problems at the second (sexuality) can influence the heart (fourth) as well as the power center (third). Everything is interrelated.

For example, just by feeling the spin of energy at the feet, you may be able to feel if that person is "walking in their own shoes" (the energy feels strong and makes a full circle from the tip of the toes down to the heel) or whether they are "walking on eggshells" or "tiptoeing around other people" (the energy feels weak and the circle centers around the ball of the foot and doesn't reach down as far as the heel). By feeling the spin of energy at each part of the body, the practitioner can discover imbalances that a person may not even be aware of. *Note: you can feel this same spin from the top or the bottom of the foot.*

When the spin is off balance, you can work with the client using a combination of skills, including speaking about issues related to this chakra. You can use light hypnosis to guide the person through childhood traumas, birth, conception, past lives, or between lives.

While doing this, place appropriate crystals on her body, make vocal tones—or encourage your client to make tones—to release or strengthen or remove energies, or use essential oils at various parts of the body. Do not expect the crystals, tones, or oils to heal by themselves (though they might); regard them as assistants, working with you to create harmony and balance in the universe and within this individual.

Through Vibrational Alignment™ and various forms of emotional release it is possible to change the energy at the chakras. For

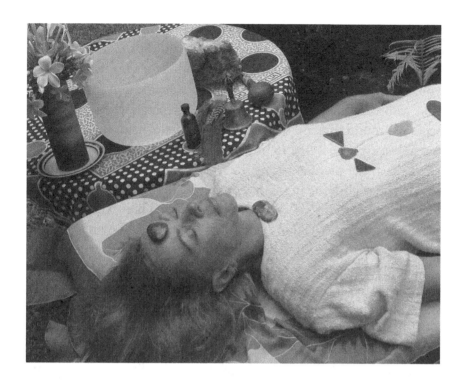

example, if a client holds resentment and pain about his mother's depression, the energy at his left hip will be blocked, which can lead to arthritis and debilitation. But if he has released his emotions about this and has forgiven and accepted his mother as she is (or was), the energy will flow unimpeded throughout his hip, and illness will not lodge there.

Always be tentative when you interpret energy. Remember that it is subjective. Do not assume that your interpretation is accurate. When you describe the energy that you feel, phrase it as a question. "The energy feels weak at your third chakra. This chakra relates to self-confidence and self-worth. Do you have any problems in this area?" Please do not say, "You've got some big problems with self-esteem."

Always honor your client. Remember that you are there to serve—not to control. Be humble. Feeling the energy is an intimate experience. A person has to be very vulnerable to allow you into his energy field. Be respectful of this.

**The Process.** Before conducting any healing process, always sit in silence for a minute. Breathe deeply and wait until to feel calm and centered. Then you can bring in white light, for both yourself and your client or friend. This involves using visualization in combination with conscious breathing to create an energetic shield of protection around the person's electromagnetic field. Here is one possible script. Feel free to improvise your own.

Take three nice deep breaths. *Pause and do this yourself.* Now inhale and feel the white light coming in through the top of your head. Bring it all the way down to your heart. Then exhale and feel it radiate into every cell of your body, pushing out any negative or stagnant energy. Feel that energy get heavy and sink down into the ground. Do this two more times. Inhale to bring the white light in and exhale to send it to every cell. Repeat.

Now inhale, bringing the white light through the crown of your head, down to your solar plexus, above your navel. Exhale and feel the white light radiating out from your solar plexus, above your navel. Exhale and feel the white light radiating out from your solar plexus, past your body, past your aura, so that you are completely surrounded by a protective shield of white light. Let's do this two more times. *Pause to do this.* All right, let's do this two more times. Inhale and bring in the white light. *Pause to do this yourself.* Exhale and radiate it out from the solar plexus. *Pause to do this.* Once again.

Now inhale and bring the white light down to your navel again, and on the exhale, let's surround us both in white light. *Pause to do this.* And finally, let's surround this room in white light. *Pause to do this.* Now we are completely protected. Only our Guides and Angels and those who mean us well may enter in through this protective white light. And yet any energy we want to release can pass from the inside out.

At this point you may wish to make your own invocation. This is not required. The purpose of an invocation is to call from your heart and invite in any guides or masters or beings from the other side that you want to come and work with you. Before I begin, I say, *I am going to do an invocation.* Please feel free to add anything that you like. It may be wise to avoid alluding to Christian or pagan deities or anything that might make your client feel uncomfortable.

My own invocation goes something like this: *Heavenly Father, Earthly Mother, those of you in the planet, the animal and mineral kingdoms who wish to be with us today. All of our own Guides and Masters and Angels—thank you for being here. I ask to be a clear channel, to facilitate _____ in whatever the next stage of his or her unfoldment might be. Thank you for the opportunity to do this good work.*

Then ask: *Is there anything you'd like to add?* Then ask: *Would you like to state your intention for this session?* Now you are ready to begin.

Stand up and hold out your arms and hands, like a big bird, with your palms toward your client. This allows you to feel the electromagnetic aura of your client from head to toe. If he gives out a lot of energy, and if you are sensitive to energy, you may feel your arms and hands being pushed back. If he is receptive to other people's energies, you may feel your arms and hands being drawn toward him. Ideally, there will be a balance between these giving and receiving energies.

You can never heal another human being unless he is ready to be healed. Every illness is a gift—an opportunity for growth, cleansing, and renewal. If we simply take away the illness, then we have deprived the person of his gift. As a true healer, your function is to work with a person, to help him grasp the nature of the challenge that his illness brings. The healing itself is not your job. Learn to "give it to God" and do not allow your ego to be attached to whether or not the healing is successful. It may be that your role is simply to help a client go peacefully to his death.

As you feel the spin of energy at the chakras you may use a combination of skills to bring balance to the chakras. You may talk about the energy and insights that come through as you correlate the energy that you feel at each chakra with your understanding of their functions. You may make sounds to describe the energy. (For example, if the energy is slow and depressed, your sounds may be slow and sad.)

If there is unresolved grief or some kind of blockage at the heart chakra, for example, you may provide an opportunity for this person to release his pain and drain his pool of sorrow. Often it is the role of the healer to simply listen, so clients can heal themselves. Use your intuitive faculties to sense which vibratory tools will help bring your client into alignment. Through the perfection of their innate being, the flowers and crystals share their energetic resonance with us; by being in their presence, we remember our own perfection.

Going from the feet to the head usually takes more than an hour. At the end of the session, go from the head back down to the feet, moving the crystal clockwise to restore the normal spin (unless this is uncomfortable for your client). During this time you are just making sure that every chakra is balanced. This is usually accomplished in a few minutes. However, if you find a chakra that is not in balance, you may want to remove the crystals in that area and replace them with new ones. More work may be required. It is not always possible to balance every chakra in a single treatment.

It is generally sufficient to feel the energy at the front of the body. But if a person has back problems, and if these problems still persist after going through all the chakras, ask her to turn over so you can feel the spin of energy at painful areas on her back (which may or may not occur at the chakra centers).

When you reach the feet, remove all the crystals and then sweep the entire aura with the hands a few inches above the body, three times from the head to the feet. This sends negative energy into the earth. Then sweep from the feet to the heart, three more times. This brings the earth energy up through the lower chakras, which helps with grounding.

You may feel inspired to sound over the person, allowing various Shamans to work their magic through your hands and voice. My clients usually go into a deep trance during this last phase. I believe this is when the sound penetrates their bodies at the cellular level, creating changes in their DNA. Some of my students have learned to do this, and others have devised different techniques that serve them well.

Then you may leave the room quietly, allowing your client to lie peacefully for five or ten minutes, to integrate the experience. (Tell her beforehand that you will do this.) When your client stands up, ask if she would like a hug, if that feels right to both of you. Then give your client an obsidian egg or a hunk of obsidian to hold onto for a few minutes, to help her get grounded before she leaves. If the client feels dizzy or disoriented, encourage her to walk outdoors for a while before driving away.

The best way to convey how Vibrational Healing works is to follow a session through from beginning to end. So I will describe a session I did recently for Lucille, an elderly woman who was experiencing senility. Lucille's daughter, Hannah, had read about me in Susanne Sims' *Healing Vacations in Hawai'i, A Travel Guide To Retreats, Alternative Healers, and Spas* (Watermark Publishing, Honolulu, 2004). The mother and daughter had been coming to Hawaii every winter for the last ten years and Hannah feared this may be their last year to make the trip together because Lucille was going downhill fast.

When Hannah called to make an appointment for herself she wasn't sure her mother would be wanting a session. "You just can't tell about her these days. One day she seems fairly coherent and the next day she can't remember a thing."

"That's all right," I reassured her, "I'll schedule her in and then we'll see how it goes."

On Monday morning the daughter and mother arrived at my door. Lucille stood there with her walker, wearing her gray correctional shoes that were in stark contrast to the simple sandals that most people kick off before entering homes on the island. Lucille's eyes had that gray overcast look so characteristic of elderly people who "aren't all there."

"It's fine to wear your shoes inside," I told her as Hannah removed her own sandals and then helped her mother to bring her walker inside. I took them both onto the lanai that looks out at a huge boulder in the backyard. I offered them cold water, and we sat and chatted as we listened to the stream that runs alongside the house and the melodies of the big wind-chimes.

Lucille stared off into the distance. I asked if she would be comfortable waiting there while I worked with her daughter. "Oh yes," she said and smiled at me courteously.

Hannah went into my office with me and she confided that she was worried about her mother. "Two years ago she was normal. We were swimming at the beach together. She's only 76. She's strong. Her sight is good, her hearing is good, her family loves her. But we seem to be losing her. Just this morning she sat by the pool for an hour by herself, talking to the imaginary fish."

I spent the next two hours doing a Vibrational Alignment for Hannah that took away her headache and gave her some powerful tools for reducing stress and helping her to sleep. Then we both went back to the lanai.

"Well, you look better!" Lucille observed, looking up at her daughter who was smiling broadly. "It's very nice out here," Lucille said to me approvingly as I sat down alongside her at the table. Before long we had established the fact that we were both Aquarians and we had both lived pretty rebellious lives. Soon we were laughing and joking.

"So, you going to do a session for me now?" she asked.

"Sure," I said, "I'd love to." Hannah and I exchanged nods and I helped Lucille bring her walker through the door and down the hall into my office. She sat down on the open futon couch and while she removed her shoes I sprayed the room with Crystal Clear, a flower remedy from Petaltones in England that clears the energy. I stepped into the bathroom and washed the stones that I used on her daughter under cold running water, dried them, and put them back on the table with the other crystals that I use for healing.

Then I sat down alongside Lucille. I told her what I would be doing during the Alignment. Then we sat in silence for a minute. I said a prayer and brought in the white light. Then I felt her overall energy. She wasn't giving out any energy at all, but she was doing okay with receiving energy. I told her that and she nodded.

I felt the spin of energy at both feet and it was very slow. She wasn't really going anywhere. She had no real enthusiasm for life.

She nodded about that too. I placed a red garnet next to each foot. Garnets are good for increasing energy and enthusiasm.

Her left knee felt okay about responsibility (the circle had an easy spin and it was reasonably energetic), but her right knee seemed a little rebellious about it (the circle was irregular in shape and slowed down in some places). She told me that she was tired of having to pay the bills and she was thinking about asking someone else to take care of that. I knew from talking to Hannah that Lucille could afford to do that. I didn't feel the need to do anything to change that energy.

The spin at her left hip was strong and healthy and had an uplifting feeling to it. "It feels like your mother had a nice energy when you were a baby. I'd say she enjoyed being a mom," I said.

"Yes, that's true," said Lucille, "she was very good to all three of us."

"That's kind of unusual," I remarked. "I noticed that Hannah received that same kind of nurturing from you when she was a baby." Lucille looked up at me with her blue eyes and it seemed like her appreciative glance pierced through some of the gray fog.

Then I felt the energy at her right hip and it was clearly evident that her father was a big man with big energy, but he wasn't always there for her. (The circle was big and energetic, and while I felt it I could literally see her father with a round face and a full beard, laughing and speaking in a robust voice—but then there were parts of the circle where the energy seemed to fall off.) I asked her if the man I saw was her father, and she nodded and smiled fondly as she thought of him. Then I asked gently if sometimes she felt as if he wasn't there for her. "Oh yes! He was a very busy man. Very active in the community. He belonged to the Masons." I put a green waterworn B.C. (for British Columbia) jade on her right hip. Jade holds the nurturing and supportive energy of the father.

The first chakra at the pubic area combines the energies of both hips. It indicates whether a person received unconditional love and affection as a child. The spin at Lucille's first chakra was strong and balanced. I told her this and she agreed.

The second chakra below the navel relates to sexuality, sociability, and desire. As I felt the spin there I felt myself going into a slightly altered state. The spin had a kind of rich texture to it. "Your family is very important to you, isn't it?"

"Yes," she responded, "my family is everything to me."

Suddenly I remembered that Hannah said that Lucille had been fine until two years before. "What happened two years ago?" I asked.

"Two years?" she said, and I could see her getting that glazed expression again. "Why do you ask?"

I decided to gamble on the truth. "Your daughter told me that was when you started losing your memory. So I'm thinking that perhaps something very traumatic happened to you then. And maybe it had something to do with your family."

"No, I can't think of anything," she said in a monotone.

"All right," I said. "We'll just go on, and maybe it will show up later."

When I got to her third chakra, the energy felt good. "You seem to feel pretty good about yourself," I said.

"Yes, I do," she remarked. "I have lived a full life. I have two beautiful children that I'm very proud of."

"Two children?" I retorted. "I haven't heard about your second child."

"Ron is a very successful businessman." She turned to look up at me. "He bought me a beautiful house on a lake outside of Seattle, and I have two young women who take care of me every day. Ron travels all over the world, but the family spends every Christmas with me." Then she raised one of her fingers. "But not the last one. Laura was there with her husband and their two boys. But Ron wasn't there."

"All right," I said as I moved the crystal to her heart chakra. The energy felt slow and weak. It felt like there was something she was avoiding. Something she was not talking about. I moved the crystal to her throat chakra and sure enough, the energy was very weak at her communication center. I felt sure it was something related to her family. Something that happened two years ago. I often feel like I'm in the middle of a mystery novel when I do this work.

"Why wasn't Ron with you last Christmas?" I asked.

"Oh, he wasn't there the Christmas before that either," she remarked casually.

"Why not?" I persisted.

"Oh, he had to have some kind of tests."

Little by little it emerged that he had cancer. He found out two years ago. But he didn't want anyone to talk about it. And especially, he didn't want anyone to cry about it. Every time she thought about it she wanted to cry. But if she cried when he was there, he would leave. She didn't want him to leave, so she didn't want to think about it or talk about it because then she would cry. But she couldn't prevent herself from thinking about it unless she just stopped thinking about everything. The rest was obvious.

I put an azurite-malachite stone at Lucille's throat, to stimulate her voice box so she would want to talk about it. Soon I would invite Hannah to come in and we could all talk about it. But first I wanted to finish the alignment. I felt the spin of energy at her forehead, and it felt strong and open. "You feel very open-minded about metaphysical type things, don't you?"

"Oh yes, ever since I was a girl I've been hearing voices."

"What kind of voices?" I asked.

"Well, after my husband died two years ago he would come back and talk to me. He still does."

"Your husband died two years ago," I reiterated. "Were you talking to him at the pool this morning?"

"Why yes!" she exclaimed. "Now young lady, how did you know that?"

"Just guessing," I smiled.

I moved the crystal up to her crown chakra. The spin felt strong and good. "Do you believe in God?"

"Yes I do. I go to church every Sunday and we have a minister that I just love."

"Do you mind if I invite Hannah to come in and talk with us?" I asked.

"Well, of course not!"

So I removed the crystals and Hannah came in and the three of us sat and talked about Ron. I urged Hannah to tell her mother everything she knew about his health, the tests he had had, the treatments he had been taking, how they both felt about his being ill, what his chances of survival were. They held each other and cried together.

I didn't even have to finish going down through the chakras. When Lucille walked out of my office she didn't use the walker. She didn't want to put on her correctional shoes. She was laughing and talking about how she was going to have to get herself some more colorful clothes to wear. She was bored with all those beige suits she'd been wearing.

I got an email from Hannah a few months later. She thanked me profusely for the work that I did with her and with her mother. Hannah didn't need sleeping pills anymore. She admitted that her sleeplessness had been related to her inability to talk about her concerns about her brother. Now that she and her mother could talk openly about it and could cry openly about it they were better able to cope with their grief. They both hoped that Ron would come and see me. Eventually he did, but that is a story for my next book.

## Feeling Your Own Chakras

Lie on your back and pass your hand over your front midline, from the pubic area to the top of your head, a few inches above your body. As you pass over each energy center, you may feel them as intense concentrations of energy. Try doing this with your right hand and then with your left. You may see the colors of the chakras with your inner sight, even if you aren't looking directly at them (it may be easier to do this with your eyes closed) because you are using inner vision.

Move your hand in a circular motion above each chakra, and pay attention to what you feel. Does the energy seem to change? Do you feel a warm or a cool sensation? Does the energy seem to stop or does it flow freely? Do you get any visual impressions or bodily sensations while you are at a given chakra?

You can use colored pens to draw your chakras and you can write in a journal about the impressions you receive at each chakra.

# PART 2

# Light, Color, and Frequencies

When you are born, you move out of darkness and into light. The Hopi used to keep the newborn in darkness for twenty days. Then the infant would be taken outdoors and held up to her Divine Father, the Sun.[1] By contrast, most of us begin and end our lives in sterile hospitals, under bright glaring lights, offensive antiseptic smells, and the blaring sound of a television.

There was a time when you lived in a watery darkness, gently nurtured by muted frequencies. The rhythmic contractions of your mother's uterus ushered you toward the light, where you disconnected from the familiar rhythms of your mother's heart and blood, and took on the unique sound signatures that would accompany you through every moment of the rest of your life.

What could be more profound than this movement out of darkness, into the particular frequency of sound that still holds you in the unique shape and form that you recognize as your body? Every sound you hear comes through the filter of the three primary sounds of your nerves, muscles, and blood. Everything you see comes through the rose- or other-colored glasses of your electromagnetic aura.

## Science of Electromagnetism

It's plain to see that your body is made up of solid flesh, blood, and bone. You know that hormones and chemicals affect the function of your body, so it's not hard to grasp that drugs (pharmaceutical or otherwise) affect your emotional and physical well-being. But how can light, color, sound, or smell affect your emotions and even alter the structure of your body?

I do not expect you to take a huge leap of faith into the world of Vibrational Healing. I will not ask you to leave your mind behind. When you fully grasp how *unsolid* your body really is you will appreciate how the vibrations of your body are highly mutable and fully capable of entraining to the healthy balanced frequencies of nature, as experienced through light, sound, color, aromas, and crystalline structures.

The following section describes the language of waves and frequencies so you can better understand the world of vibrations. It is not essential to read this section to use the tools of Vibrational Healing, but it will give you a greater understanding of how they work. If you are a healer, you will feel more confident and better able to explain the process to others.

This section is highly technical, so if you are not scientifically inclined, you may find it challenging. If you read it once quickly and then return later and read it again, you will be amazed at how much easier it becomes the second time.

Once you comprehend the basic nature and language of vibrations, you can appreciate how—under the best conditions—natural forces feed your vibratory field. You will learn how human-made devices alter your vibratory field—both positively and negatively. While vibratory tools can help offset the negative effects of destructive force fields, it is far better to avoid exposure in the first place. By educating yourself about healthy and unhealthy environments you can add many years to your life.

## The Electromagnetic Spectrum

Electromagnetic radiation is a mixture of radiation of different wavelengths and intensities. The electromagnetic spectrum includes, in order of increasing frequencies: electrical power and telephone waves, television and FM waves, microwaves, infrared light, visible light, ultraviolet light, X-rays and gamma rays, and cosmic rays.[2, 3] (*See illustration.*) These different forms of energy have a direct impact upon your health, but most people are ignorant about their effects, because the majority of these frequencies

# ELECTRO MAGNETIC SPECTRUM
## IN HERTZ FREQUENCIES

Not to Scale

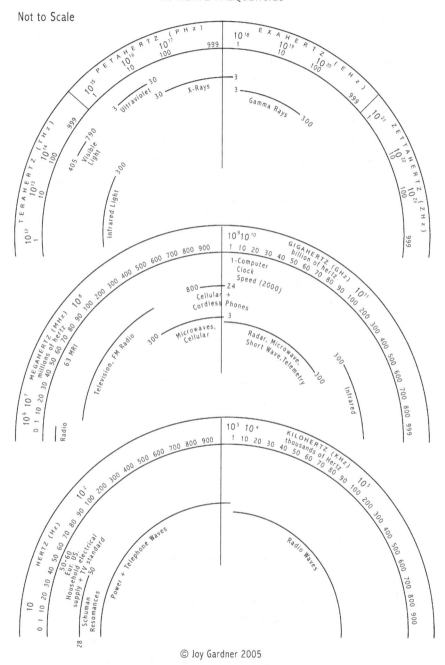

© Joy Gardner 2005

are invisible. By taking the time to learn about their effects you can empower yourself to choose which frequencies to bring into your body, and to what degree.

The Electromagnetic Spectrum can be confusing because different sources are measured in different units. The wavelength distribution is vast, so it is impossible to put all the sources on one chart, according to scale. The length of a cosmic ray is as short as 0.0000000000003937 of an inch, and the length of an electric wave can be as long as 3,100 miles![4] Clearly it would be too tedious to state the multiple fractions of an inch for 3,100 miles.

Electromagnetism is defined as the physics of electricity and magnetism. Electrical energy flows throughout the body and is produced by the body. Magnetic fields operate within and around the body.[5]

The magnetic field of the sun increases one hundred to one thousand times during increased sunspot activity, affecting both the magnetic and electrical fields of the earth and its atmosphere.[6]

Scientist Valerie Hunt conducted experiments that help explain how electromagnetism affects the human body. In one experiment she monitored subjects in the Anechoic Room at UCLA where a group of four individuals experienced a field devoid of electromagnetic energy, where sound and light were completely blocked. "Immediately we felt strange sensory aberrations; we lost the sense of time. . . our consciousness altered so rapidly that we were unable to operate instruments."

Then a group of subjects was taken to a small shielded room in the physics department where the natural electromagnetic frequencies could be altered without changing the level of gravitational force or the oxygen content in the room. When the electrical energy was diminished, participants were unable to identify the locations of their bodies in space.

"The subjects burst into tears and sobbed, an experience unlike these people had ever endured. Although they reported that they were not sad, their bodies responded as though they were threatened, as they might be if the electromagnetic environment which nourished them was gone. Any sense of body boundary, the body image was absent. . . ."

When the electrical field was increased above normal, the subjects' thinking became clear, and they had a sense of consciousness expansion. When the electrical level in the room remained normal but the magnetism was decreased, the subjects became uncoordinated and lost kinesthetic awareness. Their sense of balance was thrown off, and they had difficulty doing simple tasks such as touching a finger to a nose.

When the magnetic field was increased beyond normal, the subjects displayed extraordinary motor coordination and balance. Dr. Hunt deduced that a normal electromagnetic environment is conducive to carrying out physiological processes and to having normal emotional experiences. An advanced level of electromagnetism improves motor performance, emotional well-being, and a sense of higher consciousness. A diminished level of electromagnetism results in lower motor, sensory, and intellectual abilities as well as increased anxiety and emotion.[7]

Many authorities tell us the electromagnetism of our planet has been steadily decreasing and is currently at an all-time low. So it is not surprising that people are experiencing phenomenal amounts of anxiety, depression, and learning disabilities. Any way that you can bring higher levels of electromagnetic energy into your life will help counterbalance this effect. Spending more time outdoors in nature is one way to do this. Bringing more light, color, sound, essential oils, and crystals into your home, school and office will increase the electromagnetic energy, uplifting spirits, making it easier to concentrate, and creating a better sense of bodily awareness.

## Terminology of Waves and Electromagnetism

The world of vibrations includes sound, light, and even aromas, yet they seem to be entirely different spheres. By understanding the terminology of waves and electromagnetism, you will see how they are all interconnected. **Frequency** is measured according to the number of oscillations or **cycles per second (cps)** of a wave (*see figure A*). Frequency is measured as **Hertz (Hz)**, the number of cps at which energy moves in a cyclical form. Each oscillation is a complete wave cycle, including the rise and fall of the wave.

Figure A.
Hertz Frequencies

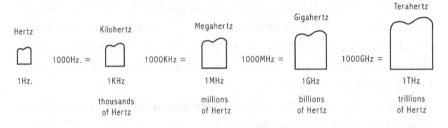

frequency = the number of oscillations of waves per second

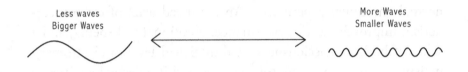

**Hertz frequencies** are used to measure the rates of events that happen periodically in a fixed and definite cycle. The unit is named after German physicist Heinrich Rudolf Hertz (1857–1894), who demonstrated in 1887 that energy is transmitted through a vacuum by electromagnetic waves. The **becquerel** also equals one event per second and is used to measure the rates of things that happen randomly or unpredictably.

**Wavelength** is the distance from one wave crest to the next (*see figure B*). The higher the frequency, the shorter the wavelength. The length of a wave is measured in nanometers (nm), each of which is one thousand millionth of a meter. A meter is close to a yard in length at slightly less than 40 inches. A nanometer is actually about the length of two atoms.

A complete oscillation is a complete wavelength. Objects are said to be oscillating when they move in regular, repeated cycles. The period of an oscillation is the length of time it takes to complete one full cycle. If the crest of one ocean wave hits the shore every two seconds, the period of oscillation is two seconds. Since frequency is the number of cycles completed per unit of time, the wave would be moving at two cps.

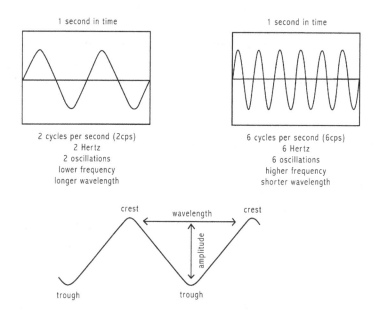

Figure B.
Putting Waves in a Box

1 second in time

2 cycles per second (2cps)
2 Hertz
2 oscillations
lower frequency
longer wavelength

1 second in time

6 cycles per second (6cps)
6 Hertz
6 oscillations
higher frequency
shorter wavelength

crest  wavelength  crest
amplitude
trough  trough

The top of each wave is called the **crest** and the bottom is called the **trough**. The distance from crest to trough is the **amplitude**. The speed at which the wave travels is the **velocity**. The greater the amplitude of a wave, the more energy it carries. Loud sounds (like those made by ocean waves crashing against cliffs on the shore) are made by high-amplitude waves with lots of energy. The amplitude of sound diminishes drastically as the sound wave travels because the wave spreads out in three-dimensional space instead of traveling in a single line along a one-dimensional medium.

Electromagnetic energy and sound waves are always confined to the constraints of a constant speed. This is like putting a wave of a given length in a box that represents a second in time. (*See figure B.*) The length of an electromagnetic wave within the box is a constant 186,000 miles, so it takes one second for a wave of light to travel 770 miles. The wave inside a box can open up and stretch itself out into two long, slow oscillations (the equivalent of 2 cps or

Hz), or it can curl itself up, for example, into six fast little impulses (the equivalent of 6 cps or Hz).

A crude but memorable metaphor is to compare the wavelength to a woman's hip measurement. You can have three broad women standing side by side in a closet (akin to the left side of the EM spectrum), or you can have six skinny women standing side by side in the same closet (akin to the right side of the EM spectrum).

Now I haven't said anything about the height of the women (or the waves). They will all be the same height as each other. When you adjust the amplitude, this will cause the women (or the waves) to grow taller or become shorter. The more amplitude, the stronger the waves. In this metaphor, the tall women will be more forceful. Changes in amplitude account for a weak or strong radio signal, greater or lesser volume, and dim or bright lights of the same color.[8]

An excellent interactive website at http://micro.magnet.fsu. edu/primer/java/wavebasics allows you to adjust different frequencies and watch how increasing the frequencies (more waves) automatically diminish the length of waves (more skinny women). Decreasing the frequencies (less waves) automatically increases the length of the waves (less broad women). Frequency and length of the waves change in inverse ratio to each other. When amplitude or energy is added or subtracted, the number and width of each wave remains the same, but the height of the waves increases or diminishes.

Since the terminology of sound and light are different, the measurement of light or photons is in nanometers, and the measurement of sound is in hertz frequencies. Light waves are measured primarily by frequency. By using mathematical language we cab measure light in hertz frequencies, which enables us to grasp the vibrationary connection between sound and light.

## Visible Light: Frequencies of Colors

The narrow band of light visible to the human eye comprises just 2 percent of the electromagnetic spectrum. Light that is invisible to humans has wavelengths that are longer and slower (infrared) and shorter and faster (ultraviolet) than the human eye can see. However, the body can *feel* the warming rays, and the skin can experience the penetrating ultraviolet rays of the sun, which (in excess) can cause sunburn.

We think of the color spectrum as red, orange, green, blue, indigo, and violet, but there is actually a continuous blending of colors from red to violet. The colors are usually measured in nanometers. The length of a wave of violet light is about 380 to 440 nm; indigo (a puplish blue) is 440 to 485 nm; blue or cyan is 485 to 500; green is 500 to 565; yellow is 565 to 590; orange is 590 to 625; and red is 625 to 740 nm.

The colors of light can also be measured in Hertz frequencies, using trillions of Hertz (THz). As the wavelength increases, the frequency decreases, so moving from violet to red, the numbers grow smaller instead of larger. The frequency for violet light is about 790 to 680 THz; indigo is 680 to 620; blue is 620 to 600; green is 600 to 530; yellow is 530 to 510; orange is 510 to 480; and red is 480 to 405 THz. This means that you look at the color red, your eyes receive more than four hundres trillion waves per second.[9]

Electromagnetic waves move in a stream of particles or energy packets called *photons*. All the energy packets of a given color have the same amount of energy. So all the energy packets of red light are the same size, and all the energy packets of violet light are the same size. The red energy packets are relatively small, and the violet ones are relatively large.[10]

Photons have no mass, but frequencies associated with the color red have a longer wavelength than the other colors. (*See figure C.*) Red can be seen on the left of the range of visible light, and violet is at the right. As you move from left to right, you move from lower Hertz with relatively low frequency to progressively higher Hertz, with relatively high frequency.

I used to find this confusing because I thought of red light as having high energy and being hot and penetrating, so I imagined that the red end of the spectrum would have lots of small, fast waves, and the violet end of the spectrum would have cool, slow, big waves.

In fact, as you move past the violet end, you move into the invisible rays of ultraviolet, and then X-rays and gamma rays. As the wavelengths become smaller, they become so tiny that they easily penetrate the skin, causing burns and possibly cancer. As you move in the other direction, past the red end of the spectrum, you find the slow, invisible, warming, and healing rays of infrared.

Returning to the metaphor of the women in the closet, you could dress the broad women in red and dress the thin ones in violet, and you would have a pretty good visual.

Color is a subjective experience, governed by the eye. A person who is color-blind sees different colors than a normal person. There are just three color-sensitive cone cells in the retina, and each has a pigment that is sensitive to a specific range of wavelengths of light. Under normal lighting conditions, the color you see depends on the degree to which each pigment is stimulated.

When you see a leaf as green, the chlorophyll is reflecting green light and the leaf is absorbing all the other colors. Black has no

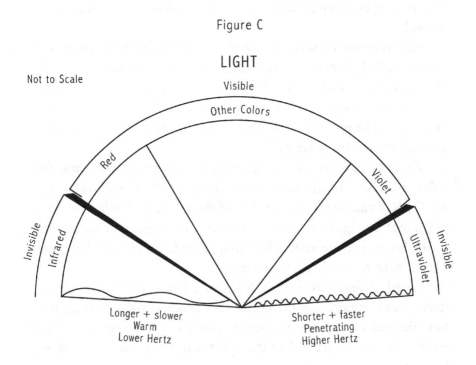

Figure C

LIGHT

Not to Scale

Visible

Other Colors

Red

Violet

Invisible

Infrared

Ultraviolet

Invisible

Longer + slower
Warm
Lower Hertz

Shorter + faster
Penetrating
Higher Hertz

color, so it absorbs all of the light rays. White has all colors, so it bounces off all of them.[11] The usual interpretation is that the leaf contains everything *except* green. I disagree. We interpret chlorophyll as green. The leaf already has an abundance of green, so it reflects that color because it doesn't need it. Therefore that color or wavelength or frequency becomes available for us to see and use.

Light is seen as white when all three cone cells of the eye are stimulated by equal amounts of red, green, and blue light. These are the primary additive colors. When the red and green cone cells are stimulated equally, you see yellow (the complement of blue). Red and blue yield magenta (the complement of green), and green and blue result in cyan (the complement of red). Cyan is in the range of 600 to 620 THz. Since those two red and blue are at opposite ends of the natural spectrum, magenta does not appear in the color spectrum at all. The screen of a color TV or a computer monitor contains a combination of just three kinds of dots: red (long wave), green (medium wave), and blue (short wave). This is the additive color system, and when you start with a black surface and add all three colors you get white.[12]

In the subtractive system used for almost all printing and painting the primary colors are red, yellow, and blue. You start with a white surface, like a piece of paper, and add different amounts of red, yellow, and blue. With a printer you add cyan, magenta, and yellow.[13]

In psychic healing, when you visualize removing something from the body, it is common practice to put it into the violet light, which is supposed to dissolve it into free atoms. I've always thought of violet light as being in that gray zone where something becomes so extreme that it changes into its opposite (the Chinese would say that yin changes into yang, or vice versa). Perhaps it would be more accurate to suggest that we put such objects into the magenta light.

## Invisible Light

Sunlight begins in the invisible infrared band, ranging from 700 nm to 1 mm. The length of these waves is longer than visible light. When sunlight moves into the invisible ultraviolet range (180 to 380 nm), wavelengths become so tiny that they are measured in electron volts (eV). An electron volt is the energy gained by an electron (or proton, which has the same amount of electric charge) moving through a voltage difference of one volt.

**Infrared Light.** In 1800 the astronomer Sir William Herschel was trying to understand why different filters on his telescope seemed to heat up differently. Herschel separated sunlight into its spectrum with a prism and then used three thermometers with their bulbs blackened with soot. He put one bulb in each color of the spectrum, and he used the other two bulbs as controls. He found that each color of light produced a temperature higher than the controls, and the temperature increased as he moved from the blue to the red. When he measured the temperature just beyond the red, he discovered a region where no visible light produced the highest temperatures. Herschel correctly surmised that there was a portion of light beyond the red, which we now call infrared.[14]

Cameras mounted along a highway can take your picture with an infrared light beamed into your car at night. You won't see the light, and you won't know the picture was taken. Infrared light can be used to map the dust between stars. Some animals, like the pitviper, have infrared detectors that enable them to find their prey in the dark. Infrared has a longer wavelength (less energy) than regular red light. The infrared portion of sunlight transmits warmth to the skin. Every warm object emits infrared electromagnetic radiation.[15]

**Ultraviolet Light.** Ultraviolet radiation ranges from about 3 to 100 eV. Ultraviolet's short wavelength gives off more energy and is more penetrating than visible light, which is why it can cause sunburn and skin cancer when absorbed in excess. Honeybees see this light, and certain flowers that appear white to us may appear multi-hued to the bees.

Ultraviolet light stops abruptly at 290 nm. Beyond this intensity, its rays cannot penetrate the earth's atmosphere, and they can only be detected by devices located outside of the earth's atmosphere. There are three categories of UV light:

**Near Ultraviolet (320 to 380 nm):** These long and apparently harmless wavelengths penetrate the earth's atmosphere at intensities akin to visible light, including black light ultraviolet, which gives unusual lighting effects.

**Middle Ultraviolet (280 to 320 nm):** Middle-range wavelengths, also known as tanning ultraviolet light, are classed as UVB. This range has strong potential for burning and damaging skin, even at fairly low intensities. Sources emitting UVB should not be used for illuminating skin except under carefully designed and controlled conditions, such as therapeutic exposures and tanning facilities, where adequate distance between the light and skin is maintained, time of exposure is controlled, and eyes are protected.

**Far Ultraviolet (180 to 280 nm):** These shorter wavelengths include the germicidal wavelengths that can be very harmful. Stars and other "hot" objects in space give off far UV radiation.[16]

## Other Forms of Electromagnetic Energy

**Radio Waves.** Most of the radio part of the electromagnetic spectrum occurs between 1 kilohertz (KHz) and 1 megahertz (MHz). Radio waves comprise a very broad band of the spectrum.[17] They have a lower frequency and longer wavelength than light waves, ranging from about ten feet to many miles in length. Radio waves are continuous.

Radio waves are emitted by radio stations and also by stars and gases in space. Radio telescopes can penetrate the earth's atmosphere even on cloudy days, and two telescopes can pick up fine detail of the entire distance between them.[18]

**Microwaves or Millimeter Waves.** Millimeter radio waves, also known as microwaves, range from around 300 million waves per second (300 MHz) to 3 billion waves per second (3 GHz).[19] Their wavelength is about 1 inch long. Microwaves are used in microwave ovens because the energy is converted into heat and is easily absorbed by water, making the water molecules vibrate faster.[20]

Microwaves are used in radar. Millimeter waves are used in telemetry in space programs. Scientist Valerie Hunt used them to measure the human energy field (see Light and the Human Energy Field, page xxx). Microwave transmitters, including those that power cell phones, need to be in sight of each other. Each antenna is a half-wave long, no more than a couple of inches, is backed up by a parabolic dish that reflects the waves into a narrow beam to the next tower.[21]

As you become increasingly aware of the power of vibrations to affect your health, it becomes self-evident that vibrations also have the power to make you sick. Mobile phones and even cordless phones operate on frequencies that are potentially dangerous to the body. As the waves (hertz) get smaller and faster they become increasingly penetrating.

After radio waves, the next smallest are X-rays. When I was a kid, every good shoe store had an X-ray machine where you could look at your feet inside the shoes. As we became more knowledgeable, it became apparent that such machines were outright dangerous and their use was discontinued.

From 1953 to 1976, the Soviets directed microwave radiation at the U.S. embassy in Moscow from the roof of an adjacent building. When the embassy staff heard that this could lead to health problems, they researched the health effects of microwave exposure. Most of the information was found in Soviet literature, and it indicated adverse health effects in lab animals and individuals working with radar. Most microwave-related symptoms were psychological, including lethargy, lack of concentration, headaches, depression, and impotence. Soviet medical journals termed this syndrome "microwave sickness." The Soviet safe standard for microwave exposure is more than 100 times lower than the American recommendation."[22]

**X-rays.** X-rays are another form of electromagnetic radiation with high energy and short wavelengths, ranging from 100 to 100,000 eV or 100 eV to 100 KeV. The extremely high-energy radiation found in X-rays and gamma rays is produced by particles moving at very high velocities (speed of motion), which produces great heat. X-rays are even more penetrating than UV light, easily passing through human skin, muscle, and tissue, but not through calcium in bones. Hot gases in space also give off X-rays. When X-rays interact with matter, they produce ionizing radiation, which can cause mutations or cancer in tissue.[23]

Gamma-rays. All photons with energies greater than 100 KeV are considered gamma rays. These rays have the shortest wavelength (about thirty times the diameter of the hydrogen atom) and the highest energy and frequency. They can penetrate metal and are used to detect tiny cracks in airplane wings, and for radiotherapy, a therapeutic treatment that destroys cancer cells. Natural or man-made radioactive materials emit gamma rays, as do nuclear power plants and big particle accelerators.[24]

## Joy Gardner's Spectrum of Biological Frequencies

We rarely think of the body as a source of electrical energy. Yet we know that the heart gives off an electrical charge that can be measured by an electrocardiogram (EKG) at about 225 cps. Since the definition of one Hertz is 1 cps, the frequency of the human heart is about 225 Hz.

Brain wave activity is measured by an electroencephalogram (EEG) oscillating from 0 to 200 cps, or 0 to 200 Hz. When muscles tense or shorten, they produce an electrical impulse that is measured by an electromyogram (EMG) with a range from 0 to 250 cps or 0 to 250 Hz.[25]

A fundamental measurement in particle physics is known as Planck's constant. It was defined in 1900 by German physicist Max Planck (1858–1947) who showed that, at atomic and subatomic levels, energy occurs in discrete packets called quanta. Each quantum (singular for *quanta*) has energy $hf$, where $f$ is the frequency of the radiation as measured in $h$, Hertz.

Since all forms of matter are composed of atomic and subatomic particles it is safe to say that *everything vibrates*, and can be measured in Hertz frequencies.[25] German biophysicist Dr. Fritz-Albert Popp (born 1938), developed highly sensitive equipment

# Joy Gardner's
## SPECTRUM OF BIOLOGICAL FREQUENCIES

Not to Scale

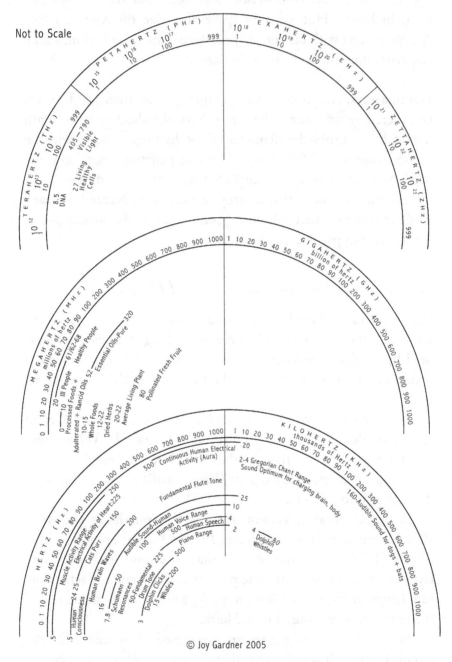

© Joy Gardner 2005

that shows that all living cells emit electromagnetic waves which produce a permanent weak light in visible range (400 to 800 nm) called biophoton emission. If the cells are healthy, they emit more; if not they emit less.[26]

The electromagnetic spectrum (see illustration on page 53) shows the range of visible and invisible light, yet I wondered why it did not show the frequencies of audible and inaudible sound. I understand now that all electromagnetic energy moves at the speed of light (186,000 miles per second), and the speed of sound is a mere 46,200 miles per second. Light is usually measured in nanometers (the length of the wave), and sound is usually measured in Hertz (the frequency of the wave, or how many waves exist within one unit of time). By measuring in Hertz frequencies, you can grasp the vibrational connection between sound and light.

Then I discovered that *smell* could also be measured in Hertz frequencies. Bruce Tainio, who invented the BT3 Monitor to measure the frequencies of plants, found that the same machine could be used to measure the frequencies of essential oils, food, and human beings.

Another term for vibrations is waveforms, which brings us to French mathematical genius, baron Jean Baptiste Joseph Fourier (1768–1830), who invented a type of calculus. Fourier developed a mathematical way of converting any pattern, no matter how complex, into a language of simple waves, then back into the original pattern. These equations are known as Fourier transforms. They are used in Fourier frequency analysis (see Science of the Chakras, page 24) and are an essential part of laser technology (see Lasers, page 74).

Fourier discovered that the visual cortex does not respond to patterns; it responds to the frequencies of waveforms. He explored the other senses and found that a hundred years previously German physicist Hermann von Helmholtz demonstrated that the ear is a frequency analyzer.

More recent research reveals that the sense of smell is apparently based on something called osmic frequencies. Georg von Bekesy (1899–1972), an American biophysicist born in Hungary, demonstrated that the skin is sensitive to frequencies of vibration, and even produced evidence that taste may involve frequency analysis. He found that physical movements are stored in the brain through a process akin to Fourier mathematics where they are converted into waveforms.[27]

Human chauvinism makes us think that reality can be defined only by what human beings experience with their five senses. It is difficult for us to believe that there are sounds we cannot hear and vibrations we cannot feel. Yet we all know that dogs and cats hear sounds that we cannot hear.

Armed with all this information, I began to imagine a spectrum that would include the range within which humans (and other animals) can see, hear, smell, taste, touch, and feel. I pondered these ideas for several years, and then I produced a Spectrum of Biological Frequencies that includes all the reliable measurements I can find thus far that relate to human and animal senses (see illustration). As I said earlier, the electromagnetic spectrum includes both frequency and wavelength. The electromagnetic chart only shows frequencies of electromagnetic phenomenon. My Spectrum of Biological Frequencies gives frequencies for light as well as sounds, aromas, and food values that we (and other animals) are capable of perceiving. I expect this spectrum to evolve over the coming years, and I invite anyone who has additional information to contact me through my website (see Resources).

Let's review the Hertz frequencies:

I Hz (hertz) = I cycle per second (cps)
I KHz (kilohertz) = I thousand cps
I MHz (megahertz) = I million cps
I GHz (gigahertz) = I billion cps
I THz (terahertz) = I trillion cps

Now let's turn to the Spectrum of Biological Frequencies on page 66. As you look at this chart, it becomes evident that we live in a sea of vibrations. By learning how to enhance or diminish the vibrations of your own body (brain, heart, muscles, and aura) through the conscious use of highly vibratory tools (sound, essential oils, and colored light), you can maintain your balance and health. This is the essence of Vibrational Healing.

If the page were longer, I would have one continuous spectrum going from 1 Hz to 1,000 GHz. Since this was not possible, I created a spectrum in three tiers, beginning at the bottom left and ending at the top right. Please note that this spectrum is not drawn to scale. It would be spatially impossible to show hertz, kilohertz, megahertz, and so forth in 10 Hz increments from 0 to 1000. Instead I have settled for going in 10 Hz increments from 10 to 100, and then leaping up to 100 Hz increments from 100 to 1,000.

## Brain Frequencies and the Schumann Resonance

Currently recorded human brain waves, as measured by an EEG, range from 0.5 to 200 Hz. The bands that define states of consciousness traditionally begin at 0.5 and go to 30 Hz.

Your normal waking consciousness, when you are engaged in an active conversation or highly alert, is generating **beta** waves, from about 40 to 15 Hz. It is also good for open focus meditation used in Zen Buddhism in which the focus is on everything simultaneously. As you become more relaxed and receptive, your brain waves become slower and higher in amplitude and you drop into **alpha** at 9 to 14 Hz. This is a time for reflection, meditation, and nonlinear, intuitive thinking.

The next level, at **theta,** from 5 to 8 Hz gives access to the subconscious where deep meditation, hypnosis, visualization, shamanic activity, and healing occur. It can also kick in while doing repetitive tasks such as running, weaving, spinning, or driving long distances. Original creative inspiration is often born while in theta and is also associated with going out of body (astral travel). This is the region of sleep characterized by active dreaming and rapid eye movement (REM). Finally, the high-amplitude, low-frequency **delta** brain waves, from about 0.5 to 4 Hz, occur during deep restorative sleep as well as profound meditation and hypnosis. In reality all four types of brain waves are always present, but only one type will predominate at any given time.[28]

The Monroe Institute in Faber, Virginia, developed a technology called Hemi-Sync using stereo headphones or speakers to deliver, for example, a sound of 300 Hz into one ear and 30 Hz into the other. The brain integrates the two signals, producing a sensation of a third sound called the **binaural beat**. The brain waves entrain or lock onto and follow the 30 Hz signal that is perceived in the bone structure of the inner ear, causing the brain to shift into high alpha or even theta brain states that are used for enhancing creativity and lucid dreaming.[29]

Studies at the Center for Neuroacoustic Research, using special equipment, have shown brain wave frequency patterns as slow as one quarter cps with patients who were experiencing extraordinary states of consciousness, including high Yogic states of suspended animation. These deepest below-delta states are called **epsilon** states. During these times the right-left hemispheres tend to synchronize as the answer to a problem or a moment of great inspiration occurs.

There is yet another phenomenon reported by other researchers in which brain wave patterns go from 40 to as high as 100 Hz or more, known as gamma brain waves, with the significantly high range being hyper-gamma. These are characterized by experiences of bringing information from all the senses together for a higher-level awareness of unity, as seen during shamanic and mystical experiences. There are even ecstatic states of consciousness recorded at frequencies of 200 Hz, called **lambda** brain wave states.[30]

From a different perspective, experimental physicist Bob Beck recorded the brain waves of proven mystics while they were doing their work and found that they vibrated at 7.8 cps, which is between theta and alpha. His work on earth resonances and their effect on brain wave frequencies was presented at a psychotronic conference in the United States and published in the late 1970s.

The earth's atmosphere, between its crust and the ionosphere, has a basic frequency of 7.83 Hz. When thunderbolts of lightning strike the earth, they travel at the speed of light, which is 186,000 miles per second. Lightning can circle the circumference of the earth exactly 7.83 times in one second, thereby imparting a 7.83 Hz charge to the earth.

About 1000 lightning storms occur every second worldwide, and collectively account for the measured current flow in the earth's electromagnetic "cavity," between the surface of the earth and the inner edge of the ionosphere, sixty-five miles above the earth. They are not caused by anything internal to the earth, its crust or its core. They are related to atmospheric electrical activity, which does increase during times of intense lightning activity and increased solar sunspot cycles that occur every eleven years.

W. O. Schumann, a German physicist, predicted and then detected these waves during the mid-1950s. He said this resonance was between 7 and 8 cps. Bob Beck found it to be 7.8 Hz, within 1/500 of a cycle.[31]

In the 1960s, this frequency was monitored by the National Bureau of Standards in Boulder, Colorado. It found that several frequencies between 7 and 50 Hz actually compose the **Schumann Resonances**, starting with a 7.8 Hz nominal figure and fluctuating in approximately 5.9 Hz progressing overtones (7.8, 13.7, 19.6, etc.). These frequencies vary from one geologic location to another, and they sometimes have naturally occurring interruptions.[32]

There is a rumor in esoteric circles that the resonance of the earth has recently increased from 7.8 to 9 Hz. I have not been able to find any reliable sources to confirm this, nor does it seem possible unless the circumference of the earth or the speed of light changed. There is also a belief that this would indicate a rise in human awareness. Actually, since the 7.8 frequency is located just at the top of theta (deep meditation and shamanic activity) bordering on alpha (normal meditation and daydreaming), a frequency of 9 would pull us *down*, out of theta entirely, and just into alpha, which would actually be a drop in human consciousness.

Valerie Hunt speculates that when mystics attune to the 7.8 Hz frequency, they gain access to all the memories of the earth and the creatures that inhabit it, including possible information from the past and future. Mystics speak about the *Akashic Records*, a psychic library where all events that have occurred on the planet are stored.

If such a channel exists, it would help explain why certain psychics can accurately *channel* information from the past and the future. I think of this channel of consciousness as being akin to the Deep Sound Channel in the ocean used by whales for communicating halfway around the world (see Sound, Science, and Medicine, page 134).

## Other Anatomical and Food Frequencies

The electrical frequency of human muscular activity begins at 0 Hz and goes up to 250 Hz, including the heart at 225 Hz. The human aura, as measured by Dr. Valerie Hunt, has a continuous radiation that begins at 500 Hz and probably goes higher than 20,000 Hz (20 KHz), but that was the highest limit of Hunt's telemetry machine.[33] DNA has been rated at 8.5 terahertz (THz or trillions of Hertz) and living healthy cells at 27 THz.[34]

According to Tainio, in collaboration with Gary Young, N.D., healthy individuals resonate in a range between 62 and 68 megahertz (MHz). This number is obtained by taking many measurements throughout the body and then finding an average. People who are ill vibrate between 20 and 62 MHz. According to measurements taken with Tainio's BT3 Frequency Monitoring System (see Resources), when you have a cold or flu your vibratory rate goes down to 58 MHz; when candida (systemic yeast infection) is present you vibrate at 55 MHz; when you have Epstein Barr virus you vibrate at 52 MHz; when you have cancer you vibrate at 42 MHz. When the death process begins, the frequency has been measured at 20 MHz.

Processed foods and adulterated and rancid oils measure from 0 to 10 MHz. It's not surprising that this kind of food is known as junk food. It has no vitality and lacks the ability to enhance your vitality. Whole foods measure from 10 to 15 MHz, and dried herbs from 12 to 22 MHz.

The average living plant is 20 to 22 MHz, and a fruit that has been pollinated can be as high as 80 MHz. No wonder raw fruits, raw vegetables, and fresh juices are so good for your health. High-quality essential oils reach an all-time high of 52 to 320 MHz.[35] No wonder you can raise your spirits, increase concentration, settle your stomach, relieve headaches, and even derive antifungal, anti-inflammatory and antibiotic effects just from smelling and applying essential oils.

## Audible and Musical Sounds

Human beings hear sounds that are in the range of 16 to 25,000 Hz (16 Hz to 25 KHz). The range of the human voice is from 100 to 10,000 Hz (100 Hz to 10 KHz). The ear is most sensitive to tones from 500 to 4000 Hz, which is also the range of normal speech. Sounds from 2 to 4 KHz are in the optimal part of the spectrum for charging the brain and body, according to Dr. Alfred Tomatis. Gregorian chants are entirely in this range.[36]

On a piano, middle C is typically 256 Hz and C an octave higher is 512 Hz (double the amount of middle C). The lowest note on a piano vibrates at 27.5 Hz and the highest at 4,186 Hz. Violins range from 200 to 2000 Hz.

Why does a violin playing the note of middle C sound different from a flute playing the same note? This can be explained by tone quality. When a violin string is bowed, it produces many frequencies at the same time. The lowest is called the fundamental, and it determines the pitch. The other frequencies are overtones, which, in the case of the violin, are simple whole-number multiples of its fundamental. The unusual tonal quality of each kind of instrument and of each instrument within that group is determined by its own mix of overtones. A flute produces a nearly pure sine wave, a pure tone without overtones. The fundamental tone of a flute resonates at 440 Hz. A drum produces its fundamental tone at 50 Hz, and its overtones have no definite sense of pitch.[37]

**Light Frequencies.** Like sound, light has a frequency and the visible spectrum of light represents about one octave (one doubling of frequency), beginning with red at 405 THz and ending with violet at 790 THz.

**Animal Sounds and Senses.** Whales and elephants make sounds between 15 and 35 Hz, so their low sounds can stimulate alpha brain activity. Southern Right whales have a discrete call used for long-range communication that has a peak energy between 50 and 200 Hz. Dolphins communicate through pulsating clicks from 3 to 500 Hz and simultaneously communicate in whistles from 2,000 to 80,000 Hz (2 to 80 MHz). The dolphin range in water is amazingly close to the human speech range in air.[38]

Dogs and bats can hear or perceive frequencies up to 160 KHz. There is a good reason why most of us find a cat's purring so comforting. House cats and wild cats purr during both inhalation and exhalation with a consistent pattern between 25 and 150 Hz, which is the ideal range for improving bone density and promoting healing. This may explain why cats purr both when pleased, as kittens do when nursing, and when in pain or under duress.[39]

## Frequencies in the Home

While the following are not actual biological frequencies, their presence in your home is likely to have an effect upon your body. In the United States, common household electrical supply is at 60 Hz, which means that the current changes direction or polarity 120 times, or 60 cps. In Europe, line frequency is 50 Hz, or 50 cps.

Most countries have chosen their television standard to match their main supply frequency. Every television picture is produced by a fast electron beam of half pictures that occur 50 or 60 times per second with a conventional 50 or 60 Hz television. That's why you see flickers when you watch carefully. Televisions are now available at 100 Hz without the flicker.

## Lasers

Nothing conveys the power of electromagnetic radiation as dramatically as the laser. It is almost impossible to grasp that light can literally cut through human flesh, weld steel, and drill two hundred holes in the head of a pin. Instead of "laser light," it would be more accurate to call it "laser radiation," since lasers use radiation of various kinds, including (but not limited to) visible light.

Laser is an acronym for light amplification by stimulated emission of radiation. The first laser was made in a microwave lasing medium, and it was called a MASER for Microwave Amplification by Stimulated Emission of Radiation.

Let us examine what these acronyms mean and how a laser works:

*1) Laser light is monochromatic—highly single colored.*

It is easier for the mind to focus on one thing in a photograph, for example, if all other distracting elements are taken out of focus. Similarly, a single bandwidth of colored light enables the eye to come into greater focus. You may notice this when you put on a pair of tinted glasses. The purer the color, the more intense the focus. You may experience this with color healing. Certain kinds of glass and plastic give a relatively pure rendition of the red frequency, for example, and this material is highly desirable when treating conditions that are responsive to pure red light, as compared to light containing elements of pink, orange, or purple.[40] A ruby crystal was used in the first laser light, because the color red is so pure.

As photographer John Ott explains, the introduction of colored filters to the microscope enabled scientists to photograph cellular materials without having to use dyes, which caused living materials to die. (Take note: artificial dyes kill cellular materials, yet we are told that food dyes are not harmful for humans. Aren't *we* made of cellular materials?) Colored filters eliminate some of the frequency bands, thus narrowing the spectrum available to the eyes.[41]

Laser light is about 10 million times more monochromatic than the best conventional laboratory light sources. The monochromatic aspect of the laser allows it to be used for highly accurate measurements. This includes measuring the position of mechanisms that store and retrieve information on computer data storage discs.

*2) Laser light is coherent—highly organized.*

Most electrons are in the lowest energy state allowed by nature. They are considered stable, because normally they will not change over a long period of time. When energy is pumped into them, they absorb the energy and become excited and move to a higher energy state. In a highly excited state they give off energy usually in the form of subatomic energy bundles of light called photons.

Different energy levels produce different wavelengths of light, and hence different colors are emitted. Without further excitation, the electrons will return to the lower energy state.

An excitation state is called quasi-stable when there are more electrons that are excited than electrons that are stable. This population inversion enables the medium to emit more light than it absorbs, thereby amplifying the light beam.

When a quasi-stable electron is exposed to another photon of light, the electron will emit another photon. This is called stimulated emission (the *SE* portion of the LASER acronym). The new photon will move in alignment with the stimulating photon. As these new photons emit more light, they excite other electrons in the lasing medium, and they all move into alignment with each other. These highly organized waves stay together in phase over long distances and long periods of time. This is called a state of coherence.

Mirrors bounce back the photons so they oscillate (swing back and forth with a steady, uninterrupted rhythm) and keep multiplying until they form a laser beam.[42]

*3) Laser light is collimated—highly directional, traveling in a narrow cone. It can maintain focus, traveling in a straight line over long distances without losing energy. It can be focused by a lens, to a point of concentration.*

Hence the use of lasers as pointers in classrooms, for measuring the distance to the moon, and for aiming rifles and satellites. A laser can be focused to a spot with a diameter nearly equal to the wavelength of the radiation.[43]

*4) Laser light is available in a wide range of power levels, from microwatts (millionths of a watt) to terawatts (million millionths of a watt). The energy is highly intense and concentrated.*

*5) Laser light is available in a continuous stream or intensely short, powerful pulses.*

Remember how, in the electromagnetic spectrum, the shorter the waves, the more penetrating, so that X-rays and gamma rays can actually penetrate the body and even metals? This explains how the short, powerful pulses of the laser are used to cut through flesh.[44]

When the laser light is divided into extremely short pulses, these are called bits. Information can be stored in digital form by turning the bits on and off. In fiberoptics each fiber carries 46 million bits per second, which allows it to transmit four thousand conversations at once. A laser the size of a grain of salt switches the bits, and another tiny laser amplifies the signal every few kilometers.

With a CD (compact disc), a much more powerful laser is used to convert music into bits that are then transmitted into the master.[45]

6) *Laser light is available in a wide range of wavelengths, including all the visible colors and X-ray lasers, microwave lasers, and even sound lasers.*

The following basic elements are needed to make a laser.

The lasing medium: This can be a gas, liquid, or solid. It must be transparent to the photons of light it produces, and it must have quasi-stable energy states so it can generate the radiation.

An excitation source: This is the laser's energy source, which may be electrical, chemical, nuclear, or optical (such as a flash lamp or another laser). This source supplies energy by causing the electrons in the lasing medium to make quantum leaps from ground states to highly excited energy states.

An optical resonator: Once the energy in a light beam is amped up, it is ready to emit optical radiation through the use of mirrors at each end of the lasing medium. These mirrors amplify the radiation of the lasing medium until there is enough energy in the beam to redirect it.

The uses of lasers are multiple. High-powered, continuous lasers can weld steel up to about an inch thick. Low-powered lasers can make very thin, precise welds. The radiation is highly concentrated at the weld, without excessive heating of surrounding material. Lasers can also be used to microsolder the microcircuits in computers and other electronic devices. Fusion is the process used by the sun to create heat. It was used in the hydrogen bomb. A highly powerful laser with light pulses of very short duration to produce fusion by heating pellets of frozen deuterium (similar to hydrogen) to millions of degrees. Fusion can also be used as a source of clean energy.

Lasers are used in surgery to make clean and highly accurate cuts that tend to bleed less because they burn the tissues (like burning the end of a rope to prevent it from fraying). Ultraviolet lasers can remove tissue by decomposing it instantly.[46]

## Cellular Response to Light and Color

The head is the receptacle of all five senses: sight, sound, smell, taste, and touch (though the sense of touch is distributed throughout the body). The pituitary gland is located deep within the center of the brain, between the right and left hemispheres. Behind and above the pituitary is the pinecone-shaped pineal gland. You can locate this gland by putting both index fingers directly behind the ears and pointing them toward the skull. It is at the center of the point where the fingers would meet if they went directly through the skull. In an adult, this gland is the size of a pea, yet its ability to absorb the life-giving rays of light can be compared to the stomach's ability to absorb the life-sustaining nutrients of food.

The pineal receives light directly from the eyes. The eyes are an extension of the brain, and electrical impulses from both the eyes and ears provide a necessary charge for the brain.[47] One function of the pineal is to register the length of daylight and night to the brain. Since the length of the days changes with the seasons, the pineal gives animals vital information about when to grow a thicker coat of fur, or when to go into heat.

The pineal gland releases the hormone melatonin in response to darkness, with a peak between 2:00 and 3:00 A.M. Approximately 100 bodily functions have daily rhythms that occur every 24 hours.[48] Swiss researchers Walter Pierpaoli and Georges Maestroni added melatonin to the nighttime drinking water of mice and found it significantly delayed or reversed the symptoms of aging, including debility, disease, and cosmetic appearance, increasing their life span by 20 percent compared to controls. They noted the progressive decline in the production of melatonin that normally comes with aging, and suggested that melatonin could be used to increase longevity, reduce stress, and help control stress-related diseases.[49]

Melatonin goes to every cell in the body. Misregulated, it can promote cancer. When regulated properly, it is a potent force for cancer prevention.[50] The pineal has a strong effect upon reproduction, growth, body temperature, blood pressure, motor activity, sleep, tumor growth, mood, and the immune system, as well as longevity.[51]

The regulation of light plays a vital role in your overall health and well-being. It has the potential to make a major contribution to your mental and physical health.

If you have ever seen a Walt Disney film where flowers magically open and pumpkins pass through their entire life cycle in a few spectacular moments, you are familiar with John Ott's time-lapse photography. Ott (1909–2000) explains in his book, *Health and Light*, that this unique method of photography requires snapping a picture once every hour for the entire life cycle of a plant, which can be as long as two years. This work has given him an opportunity to observe the profound effect that light has upon the growth of cells, plants, and animals. Through many years of study Ott became convinced that all living things require the full spectrum of sunlight in order to be healthy.

When Ott observed elodea grass under a microscope, he noticed that full natural sunlight enabled the chloroplasts (cellular structures that contain chlorophyll) to follow a typical pattern of streaming within the cells. When the cells were put under ordinary glass that filtered out the ultraviolet (UV) part of the spectrum, many chloroplasts formed a sluggish clump at one end of the cell.[52]

When Ott placed a red filter over the light, some chloroplasts continued their normal streaming pattern while others dropped out of the pattern entirely, and still others began to shortcut the pattern. When he used a blue filter, similar deviations occurred. But when he added UV light to the microscope light source, in order to more closely simulate sunlight, all the chloroplasts returned to normal patterns. Similar studies were performed at the University of Freiberg in West Germany, with comparable results.[53]

Jacob Liberman reports these same studies in his book, *Light—Medicine of the Future*. Then he speculates:

> Is it possible that cellular contortions are the microscopic equivalent of such aberrant human behavior as hyperactivity and anxiety? Could cell-wall weakening be related to breakdowns in the body's immune system? With the amount of time people spend under artificial lighting, which lacks the balanced nutritional aspects of sunlight, it may be possible that some behavioral and physiological differences among humans are in fact partially the results of their relationships to their lighted environment. . . . By spending an inordinate amount of time under artificial lights, we may be subjecting ourselves to malillumination, in much the same way as we subject ourselves to malnutrition by eating an unbalanced diet.[54]

Dr. Melyni Worth, in the *World Equine Veterinary Review*, describes experiments with tissue culture showing that visible light is absorbed by enzymes within the cell. The mitochondria (tiny rodlike structures in cytoplasm) absorb the photons of visible light, whereas invisible infrared light is absorbed by the cell membrane. We now know that cells emit and absorb light, and a lack of the full spectrum of light will eventually lead to a weakening of the cell walls.

But when infrared light is emitted—for example, through handheld portable low-level lasers—light is absorbed by the cells, and the cell membranes become more permeable, ATP levels increase making more energy, DNA production goes up, and the overall cell metabolism becomes more efficient.[55]

John Ott's work with health and light began during a time-lapse series on the growth of pumpkins for Walt Disney's *Secrets of Life*. Pumpkins have male and female flowers on the same plant. Ott attempted to grow the pumpkins under a skylight, adding fluorescent lights to mimic the full strength of the summer sun. The male flowers did well, but the female flowers turned brown and soon dropped off. When he changed to the less popular slightly bluish daylight-white tubes, the female flowers did unusually well, but the male flowers turned brown and rapidly fell off.

Ott also grew an apple for the same film and enclosed it in a glass box. Though it grew large, it remained green instead of turning red like the others. Ordinary glass cuts off 99 percent of the sun's ultraviolet radiation, so he replaced the glass with plastic that allows up to 95 percent of the UV to pass through. Within two days the apple turned red.[56]

A biology teacher approached Ott about using time lapse pictures for his fish egg research. Ott moved his equipment to the laboratory, fitting his fluorescent fixtures with cool white, daylight white, and pink tubes and suspending them over two or three fish tanks that were not located near windows. All fifty fish that hatched under the pink lights—from different parents—were female, though 20 percent of the fish later developed retarded secondary male characteristics.[57]

Meanwhile Ott developed severe arthritis in his hip. His doctor fitted him with a large metal brace, prescribed glandular extracts, which seemed to help a bit, and told him he would soon need hip replacement surgery. Ott hoped the sunlight might help his condition, so when he went to Florida for lecture engagements, he spent as much time in the sun as possible, always careful to wear his dark glasses to avoid eyestrain. He was discouraged when his condition grew worse.

He returned home and was hobbling around with a cane when he broke his glasses. The weather was warm, so while he was waiting for a new pair, he puttered around in his garden. Soon he noticed he wasn't using his cane, and he felt better than he had in years.

Ott thought the improvement might be due to being in natural daylight without his glasses, so he spent at least six hours a day outdoors, whether it was sunny or cloudy, without glasses or sunglasses. He moved his office out of the basement and into the plastic greenhouse. When he was indoors he avoided looking out of the windows, and when he was in a car he avoided looking through the windshield. He avoided bright artificial lights and did not watch television or go to the movies (this was in the days before personal computers; otherwise he would have avoided that, too). At night he used a small blue Christmas tree light as a night light in the bathroom, since he observed that turning on a bright light at night had a negative effect on some of his plants.

His arthritis improved dramatically, and he no longer needed the glandular extracts. His chronic head colds and sore throat also disappeared. But he noticed that his arthritis got worse after being under the bright studio lights during his weekly television program, or whenever he had to drive his car for a considerable distance. Ott surmised that light received through the eyes must stimulate the pituitary and/or the pineal glands, which in turn stimulated the glands that lubricated his joints.

After six months, his medical doctor took X-rays that confirmed the complete healing of a 30 percent restriction of rotation in the hip joint and a definite strengthening in the hip area. To his optometrist's surprise, Ott no longer needed the strong prisms that had previously been required to correct a muscular weakness in his eyes.[58]

Ott was careful not to draw conclusions from these singular events, but he shared his experience with a friend who followed the same regimen, and his hay fever disappeared. Another man who had been blind for four years began to spend more time outdoors, and within six months he began to distinguish colors.[59]

I can add my own testimonial. While working on this book I had been suffering for several months from a tight muscle along the outer edge of my left leg, from the buttocks to the ankle. It was aggravated from too much sitting, and was getting so bad that the outer toes of my left foot were tingling, and sometimes my left buttock became numb. I tried massage, stretches, and a visit to my chiropractor, but nothing gave prolonged relief.

After rereading Ott's book, *Health and Light*, I began spending at least two hours a day outside, or at least sitting under a full spectrum light, without my glasses. Within a week the pain and numbness were gone, and my general health was remarkably better.

The first time I read Ott's book, it was winter, and I was living in Seattle. I bought a full-spectrum fluorescent light and installed it over the kitchen sink. I never did care for washing dishes, but suddenly I found that I *wanted* to wash dishes!

In 1970 the Chinchilla Research Foundation at Utica, Illinois, completed a five-year study involving more than two thousand chinchilla ranchers throughout the world. When ordinary incandescent light was used in the breeding rooms, litters produced an average of 60 to 75 percent males. When daylight incandescent bulbs were used, litters produced an average of 60 to 75 percent females. By lengthening the hours of darkness, animals could be brought into their prime pelt season during any month of the year, rather than just in winter.

Another study, also published in 1970, showed that the number and intensity of cavities in the teeth of hamsters increased when the animals were deprived of the full spectrum of natural or simulated sunlight. Fifteen male hamsters were kept under light with added ultraviolet while another fifteen were kept under standard cool white fluorescent light. The group with the full-spectrum light averaged 2.2 teeth with cavities. On the other hand, the other group averaged 10.9 teeth with cavities that were ten times as severe. It was also observed that the development of male sex organs was only one-fifth as great in the male hamsters with the cool white light source as compared to those raised under the full-spectrum lights.[60]

Do these observations relate to human beings? I think so. When I was eight years old, my family moved from Chicago to San Diego. Some of the girls who were my age in California were already developing breasts and starting their periods. They looked far more mature than the girls in Chicago. The same is true in Hawaii where I live now.

Ott repeatedly brought his work to heads of research departments, several of whom expressed interest but confided that "participation in such an outlandish idea" would subject them to the risk of possible ridicule by other scientists. However, Dr. Jane C. Wright from Bellevue Medical Center in New York City became interested in Ott's theory about viruses, due to the belief that cancer might be caused by a virus.

When Ott demonstrated the abnormal biological effects produced in the cells by placing a blue filter in the microscope light source, two prominent virologists commented to Ott that some of those effects were similar to the characteristics of cells being attacked by viruses.

Ott tells about the problem that hothouse tomato growers had in Toledo, Ohio, when the tomato virus attacked after long periods of cloudy weather and low sunlight intensity during the short days of winter. It attacked the tomatoes even under the most sterile and carefully guarded conditions. Ott brought some of these virus-ridden tomato plants into his plastic greenhouse, and within a few days they came back to life, sending off new shoots and producing normal tomatoes.

Ott observed that "no consideration has been given to the possibility of a virus originating within the living cells of the plant itself. It seems to be generally accepted that the virus must be introduced from an outside source." He reasoned that metabolism itself is a process in which nutritional factors are fueled by light. He compared this to an automobile engine, the gasoline being akin to our consumption of food, and the spark that ignites the combustion being comparable to the sun. Just as noxious smoke and fumes can result from incomplete combustion in an engine, a poisonous chemical by-product can result from incomplete or imbalanced metabolism within the cells, due to either nutritional or light deficiency.

Such a chemical by-product would fit all the descriptions of a virus. It would not be capable of reproducing, but if injected into other cells, it might throw the metabolism of those cells off balance so they would in turn produce more of the same poisonous chemicals. The virus could be easily transmitted from one plant or person to another through direct contact or by some intermediary carrier. It could also be isolated and crystallized. It could fit all the various descriptions of a virus and still originate within the affected plant or person.[61]

Dr. Wright told fifteen of her patients with cancer at Bellevue to spend as much time as possible in natural sunlight without their glasses and without sunglasses. They were asked not to watch television and to avoid other sources of artificial light.

> According to Ott, after several months "Dr. Wright advised that while it was difficult to make a positive evaluation, it was the consensus of all those assisting in the program that fourteen of the fifteen patients had shown no further advancement in tumor development, and several showed possible improvement. The fifteenth patient had not fully understood the instructions, and although she refrained from wearing sunglasses, she continued to wear ordinary glasses during her time outdoors."[62]

When Dr. Wright attempted to pursue this further, she was criticized severely.

For his next project, John Ott partnered with his friend Dr. Samuel Lee Gabby from Sherman Hospital in Elgin, Illinois. They set up an experiment with the C3H strain of mice, which is highly susceptible to spontaneous tumor development. Thirty pairs of test mice were kept in a room under daylight white fluorescent tubes, thirty pairs were kept in a room with pink tubes, and the eight control pairs were kept in a room with daylight filtered through ordinary window glass.

The mice under the pink lights had only one or two offspring instead of the normal six to fifteen. They were the first to develop cancer. A month later the ones under the daylight white tubes developed cancer, and a full two months later the control group next to the window developed cancer. A report of this study was submitted to the *Illinois Medical Journal* but was not published, and Dr. Gabby was criticized for his participation in the project.[63] This experiment was truly disturbing, since it indicates that not only are fluorescent bulbs carcinogenic, but even just a prolonged lack of ultraviolet light can in itself be a cause of cancer.

Hyperactivity is another malady that may be related to light deprivation, as shown by a pilot project conducted in four first-grade classrooms in a windowless school in Sarasota, Florida. In two of the rooms, the standard cool white tubes and fixtures were used. In two other rooms, they were replaced with full-spectrum tubes with lead foil shields. Under the standard bulbs, some children demonstrated nervous fatigue, irritability, attention lapses, and hyperactive behavior.

With the full-spectrum bulbs, and without any drugs, the children settled down and paid more attention to their teachers. Nervousness diminished, and overall classroom performance improved. Over several months, one little boy who had been extremely hyperactive was able to sit still and concentrate and could finally learn to read.

Similar results were obtained through experiments in two California schools, which resulted in improved behavior and learning abilities. The Sarasota County Dental Society monitored the experiment and showed "a significant reduction in the number of cavities and the extent of tooth decay in the six-year molars of the children under the full-spectrum lights."[64]

John Ott draws a correlation between the hyperactive reaction to standard fluorescent lights and the reaction to artificial food flavoring and colorings discovered by Dr. Ben F. Feingold of the Kaiser-Permanente Medical Center. The Feingold Diet recommended completely eliminating all foods containing artificial flavors and colors. This diet brought about dramatic improvement in fifteen of twenty-five hyperactive schoolchildren.

Dr. Louis Pasteur discovered that he could rotate a beam of polarized light through a pure solution of naturally produced organic nutrients and the light would move both right and left. But he could not rotate the light through artificially synthesized organic nutrients.

This suggests the possibility of an interaction between wavelength absorption bands of these synthetic color pigments and the energy peaks and mercury vapor lines in fluorescent tubes. For example, two children in a family subjected to the same source of low-level radiation would react differently if one preferred to drink natural cherry or strawberry soda and the other had a liking for some artificially colored green or yellow soft drink. So a reaction or allergy to fluorescent lighting could be avoided by eliminating either the soda or the energy peaks in fluorescent tubes and other types of artificial lights.[65]

After many years of rejection by the medical and scientific community, Ott was given, in 1967, the Grand Honors Award of the National Eye Institute for making an important contribution to eye care. Loyola University in Chicago awarded him an honorary doctor of science degree.[66]

Dr. Ott's experiments with colored lights show beyond doubt that the color of a light has a profound effect on glandular and reproductive activity, cavities in teeth, and behavior that is either nurturing or aggressive. It is obvious that we are dealing with a factor that is a powerful force in health and illness.

Dr. Jacob Liberman, in *Light—Medicine of the Future*, recommends spending at least one hour per day outdoors, even in the shade or a screened-in porch, by an open window or the rolled down window of your car. If you spend time in the sun, work up to being in direct sunlight gradually. Avoid or minimize exposure to direct sun between 10 A.M. and 2 P.M.[67]

I believe that every human being needs an absolute minimum of twenty minutes per day either outdoors or under a full-spectrum light, without glasses or contacts. When it isn't possible to get outside, use a full-spectrum light. Try to install full-spectrum bulbs at your workplace and in your children's schools. The small additional expense is well worth the cost.

## Practical Applications of Light & Color

**Psychological.** We know intuitively that color has a powerful impact upon the emotions, but now we have some hard data about the powerful effect that color has on the emotions. In 1942, Russian scientist S.V. Krakov wrote about "Color Vision and Autonomic Nervous System" in the *Journal of the Optical Society of America*. By 1958 he was able to demonstrate that the color red stimulates the sympathetic portion of the autonomic nervous system and that the color blue stimulates the parasympathetic portion.

Robert Gerard confirmed these findings in 1951, demonstrating that when 24 normal adult males sat in front of a screen with red light for ten minutes, their blood pressure, arousal via palmar conductance, respiratory movements, and eye-blink frequency increased. When the participants sat in front of a screen with blue or white light, these same factors diminished. Blue increased their sense of relaxation and lessened their anxiety and hostility, while red increased their tension and excitement, as well as their levels of anxiety.[68]

Neonatal Jaundice. This condition occurs in over 60 percent of babies born prematurely. Their skin turns yellow as a result of an excess of bilirubin that can lead to brain damage or even death. Hospitals commonly expose these babies to intense blue light for several days, which brings down the bilirubin levels. Prior to discovering this treatment, infants had to undergo a complete blood transfusion.[69]

Athletes. According to a Texas university study, athletes looking at red lights experienced 13.5 percent increase in their physical strength, with 5.8 percent more electrical activity in their arm muscles, compared to other light conditions. On the other hand, a reduction in muscle strength, along with a significant reduction in violent and aggressive behavior, occurred within 2.7 seconds among prison inmates placed in small pink holding cells.

Jet Lag. Researchers at Cornell University discovered that applying blue light to the backs of the knees resets the body's internal clock, eliminating jet lag and the sleep disturbances that accompany shift work.

Interior Decoration. An executive for a paint company received complaints from workers in a blue office that the office was too cold. When the office was painted a warm peach, the sweaters came off even though the temperature had not changed.

## Light Bulbs

There are three common types of artificial light bulbs. Incandescent bulbs are the egg-shaped bulbs that screw into sockets. Their power source is a hot filament of tungsten. The light spectrum is deficient in the blue end. The bulbs have almost no UV and lots of yellow and red, with a maximum amount of infrared, which is a form of heat.

A better alternative can be found in various balanced spectrum incandescent bulbs. They use a purplish neodymium coating inside the bulb that is deficient in the yellow-green ranges. They do not contain the ultraviolet portion of the spectrum, but they do present a more balanced visible spectrum of light. For example, Chromalux bulbs are neodymium coated.

High-intensity discharge lamps (HID) produce a bright orange-red or blue light, and are used in street lamps as security lights in high crime areas.[70]

Fluorescent bulbs are filled with argon gas and mercury vapor. Cathodes at each end of a tube discharge electrons when the electric current is activated. The current moves through the mercury vapor, discharging an electrical arc that produces shortwave UV light at 2,537 angstroms. This causes the phosphor coating inside the glass tube to fluoresce, converting the invisible shortwave UV to longer wavelengths of visible light. The type of glass used in the tube allows the longer wavelengths to penetrate, but filters out the shortwave ultraviolet light. Different phosphor materials fluoresce at different wavelengths, thereby producing a variety of colors.

The light actually flickers on and off at 60 Hz, which consumes nutrients in the retina.[71] Fluorescent bulbs emit trace amounts of radiation from the cathodes (the same kind of radiation found in TV picture tubes and X-ray machines, but at lower voltages). There is also a radio frequency given off by normal fluorescent tubes. According to a Russian paper, the radio frequency from fluorescent bulbs was picked up in EEG readings of human brain waves.[72] No wonder many people feel fatigued from being around fluorescent lights.

Furthermore, Dr. F. Alan Anderson, a biophysicist with the U.S. Food and Drug Administration, expressed the belief that unshielded fluorescent lights could account for about 5 percent of the total weekly dose of radiation that each person receives. (We all receive radiation from natural sources.) In susceptible individuals, this dose may be enough to cause skin cancer.[73]

Some of the varieties of fluorescent bulbs include the following.

Cool white: Their energy peak is in the yellow-orange region of the spectrum. They are deficient in red and blue-violet.[74] In Ott's experience, this type of bulb was favored by the male pumpkin flowers but was deadly to the female pumpkin flowers.

Warm white: Similar to cool white, the warm white has a spectrum that peaks more in the yellow region.[75]

Daylight white: These bulbs give off a slightly bluish color. They were favored by the female pumpkin flowers but deadly to the male flowers.

Germicidal: These tubes are made of glass that allows the shorter UV wavelengths to penetrate. It is not coated with phosphors. They kill bacteria and, according to Ott, can be dangerous and harmful to humans.

Full spectrum: Ott assisted a lightbulb manufacturer in developing a full-spectrum fluorescent tube with added ultraviolet, which nearly duplicates the natural spectrum of outdoor sunlight. These bulbs have a lead foil shield that stops trace amounts of radiation from being emitted by the cathodes. A combination aluminum "egg crate" and wire grid screen grounds out the radio-frequency energy given off by other kinds of fluorescent tubes.[76] Other full-spectrum tubes are now available, but they don't always have the lead foil shield.

Any kind of bright light used during the night disrupts the normal function of your biological clock and suppresses the pineal gland's production of melatonin. Dr. Glen Swartwout, optometrist, recommends using a red filter over any night light, flashlight, or clock light. John Ott used a small blue Christmas tree light as a night-light in the bathroom.

In 1980, Dr. Fritz Hollwich monitored the levels of the adrenal hormones, ACTH and cortisol, in people sitting under cool-white fluorescent tubes versus the effect in people sitting under full-spectrum lights. Those sitting under the cool-white fluorescents experienced significant increases in stress hormone levels, whereas individuals sitting under the full-spectrum lights had no such increases. On the basis of the work of Hollwich and others, the cool-white bulbs are legally banned in German hospitals and medical facilities.[77]

In two studies reported in the British medical journal *Lancet*—one in London and another in Sydney, Australia—researchers found that the incidence of malignant melanomas was considerably higher in office workers than in those exposed to sunlight in relation to lifestyle or occupation.[78]

## Eyeglasses and Sunglasses

Ott persuaded several of the large plastic manufacturing companies to manufacture ultraviolet-transmitting plastic material for full-spectrum spectacle lenses and contact lenses. Sunglasses are now available in neutral gray lenses that reduce all of the light intensity, whereas many other types of sunglasses are designed to cut out all of the ultraviolet and infrared and then, depending on their color, to give a considerably distorted spectrum of wavelengths. Some gray glass does not have this continuous even spectrum.[79]

Sunglasses have UV protection because the pupil of the eye gets smaller in bright light, which is a natural protection from excess UV exposure. Sunglass tints prevent the pupil from contracting, but if the lenses do not absorb UV, the delicate tissues of the eyes actually receive more harmful UV exposure as a result of wearing sunglasses.[80]

Ott tells about a questionnaire that was given to a group of college students by a professor of psychology in which they were asked if they wore tinted contact lenses or sunglasses, and if so what color. Although it is not a statistically significant number, three students at a particular college constantly wore "hot pink" glasses. These same three were considered to be the most psychologically disturbed students in the college.

Ott recommended that they stop wearing the pink glasses. One student was on the football team, and the director of the college later wrote a grateful letter to Ott, saying that when the player changed to medium gray glasses, he "was changed from a hyper-aggressive and helmet-throwing player to a very relaxed, confident person. There was a great deal of improvement in performance."[81]

Ott gave a lecture at a dinner where he sat next to the daughter of the late Dr. Albert Schweitzer. She talked about assisting her father on the west coast of Africa. Ott inquired about the cancer rate of the people there, and she said that there was no cancer when they arrived, but it had become a problem. Ott asked if glass windows and electric lights had been installed in their homes, and she said they had not. Then he half jokingly asked her if the Africans had begun to wear sunglasses. She affirmed that sunglasses had become a status symbol in their village.[82]

Dr. Glen Swartwout, optometrist, cautions against using metal eyeglass frames. He claims that the metal short-circuits the brain's hemispheres, contributing to mental confusion, fatigue, and headaches, particularly for those with a strongly dominant hemisphere. He says that most metal frames contain toxic metals such as nickel, which can be leached out of the frame by electrolytic processes, contributing to allergic and toxic reactions.

Dr. Swartwout advises against using glasses that give 100 percent correction of the vision. "Vision that is too sharp reduces the total information flow and increases stress." The total nerve current received by the brain is dramatically affected by your lens prescription, where less seems to be better. Seventy percent of the body's sensory receptors are located in the retinas of the eyes; each retina can send as much information and electromagnetic energy to the brain as all other sensory systems combined.[83]

I read Ott's book while I was in my late twenties, and because of it, even though I am significantly nearsighted, I wear my glasses only when I actually need them. Now I have a pair of *almost* full-strength glasses that I wear for driving, and weaker glasses that I use for the computer. I never wear sunglasses unless the sun is directly in my eyes while driving.

Over the years my astigmatism and night blindness have totally disappeared. I'm far less sensitive to the sun. At age sixty, I can still read perfectly without my glasses, and my prescription is lower than it was when I was in my twenties. I was also inspired by Jacob Liberman's *Take Off Your Glasses and See*. It seems that whenever I read a couple chapters in his book, my eyes get better.

My optometrist tests for the reflectivity of the fovea at the center of the macula, which is at the center of the retina. He says that in young people this point tends to reflect light, but as people grow older there is a strong tendency for the reflectivity to diminish. Mine has actually become more reflective, indicating excellent health of the eyes, with a low risk of macular degeneration (the main cause of blindness).

## Suntan Lotion and Ultraviolet Light

Dr. Liberman recommends using *no sunscreen* if you have medium to dark skin. If you are in bright midday sun for more than thirty minutes, or if you have fair skin, consider using a sunscreen that does not contain PABA. A report by the US FDA in 1989 indicated that fourteen out of seventeen suntan lotions containing PABA (which blocks UV) can cause cancer when used in the sun. Dr. Zane Krine, in his book, *Sunlight*, claims that PABA causes genetic damage to the DNA in the skin, stimulating the production of cancer cells. He says that the fat in the lotion causes the problem.[84]

In relation to the popular belief that ultraviolet light causes skin cancer and other problems, John Ott tells about how he and his wife had dinner at a Chicago hotel restaurant called Well of the Sea, where black ultraviolet lights were installed in the ceiling. These lights were used because they caused designs on the waiters' coats and menus to fluoresce. Ott wondered if the waiters had suffered from eye problems, skin cancer, or sterility.

He returned the next day to interview the waiters and discovered that the lights had been in continual use since the restaurant opened eighteen years before, and virtually the same group of men had been working there the entire time. Their health records had been consistently excellent, even during flu epidemics when many other hotel employees were ill. The hotel manager noticed that these men were courteous and efficient, and they got along well together. There were no eye problems, and not one of them wore glasses.

Ott found similar black ultraviolet lights over some of the fish aquariums at Seaquarium in Miami, Florida. They were originally used to give fish an eerie but attractive appearance, but they seemed to solve a condition called exophthalmus, or pop-eye, caused by a virus. Fin-nipping also disappeared, and certain fish thrived that could not previously be kept in captivity.[85] The black lights are a form of UVA, which penetrates through windows and is considered harmless. UVB is the tanning form of ultraviolet light and the screening of the light is measured by the Sun Protection Factor (SPF).

Chickens were found to also benefit from ultraviolet light. It is a known fact in the poultry industry that light received through a chicken's eyes stimulates the pituitary and pineal glands, increasing egg production. For this reason lights are left on in chicken coops to simulate longer daylight hours during wintertime. A lesser-known fact is that chickens raised under full-spectrum lights live twice as long, are calmer and less aggressive, and lay more eggs, and their eggs are about 25 percent lower in cholesterol.[86]

PART 3

# Healing with Color (Chromotherapy)

*Color is where the mind and the universe meet.—Cezanne*[1]

COLOR IS SUCH A SOURCE OF JOY AND DELIGHT! NOW WE ARE beginning to appreciate how powerful colored light can be. John Ott's experiments have shown that the color of light affects something as basic and vital as the sex of your babies, and the size of their genitals—to say nothing of the health of their teeth, and their ability to be agreeable rather than hostile.

Your energy field or aura precedes you wherever you go, and all your perceptions are colored by that aura. Your ability to deeply appreciate color is an indication of how open your channels are. You may be like the person who sees life through rose-colored glasses, or the one for whom all perceptions must pass through a gray fog.

There are abundant examples of people who have reached a state of ecstasy or enlightenment, who describe their experience in terms of color.

A woman who has been told that she has just three months to live attends a workshop on death and dying, finishes all her unfinished business, and begins to live her life fully. Living one day at a time, puttering in her garden, she exclaims, "Each morning I awake with such gratitude! I sleep with the curtains open so that when I open my eyes I can see the bright-colored flowers in my window box, winking at me in the sunlight!"

A man has been fasting in the desert for seven days, with nothing to eat or drink but water. He returns home sunburned, dirty, and radiant. "The colors!" he raves. "The colors are so bee-uu-ti-ful!"

A woman gives birth at home after fourteen hours of labor. She holds up her newborn daughter, looking up with gratitude at the faces of her two midwives and her husband. "You are all so beautiful! There are bright colors all around you!"

"And around you and your baby!" smiles one of the midwives, marveling at the pink, magenta, and green lights dancing around the new mother and child.

A man has a transcendent LSD trip. He stops in the middle of a city at night, staring into the neon lights. "Man! The *colors* are out-of-sight!"

Now let's look at how your aura can "color your world." A man—we'll call him Bill—has most of his savings invested in stocks, and the market takes a huge plunge. The same day his dog gets run over by a truck and his girlfriend breaks up with him. "It's been a gray day," Bill says morosely to a friend. He has no outlet for his emotions, and he seriously contemplates suicide.

Another man, Ralph, has major investments in stock, and the market takes a huge plunge. He doesn't worry too much about it; what goes down must come up. The same day his dog gets run over by a truck. He finds the dog and lovingly buries him and cries over the grave. Later that day his girlfriend breaks up with him. In his heart, he forgives her. But when he meets his close friend that night, he suggests a game of racket ball. He allows himself to take out his anger on the ball and wins the game. At sunset he takes a walk alone. The colors of the sunset are incredibly bright, and he finds himself saying aloud, "I'm so glad to be alive!"

Life is not measured by what happens to you, but how you react to those events. When the chakras are clear and open, you are like a master of martial arts, standing totally relaxed, able to respond instantly and appropriately to whatever comes your way. You are in a state of ready alertness, totally alive and in the moment.

Contrast this with the state of fear (gray), which constricts every muscle and blood vessel, leading to a deficiency of chi (energy), so the flesh loses its healthy hue and elasticity and becomes sluggish, unable to respond.

Red is the basic color of illness. It is the color of infection, repressed anger, fever, and overexertion. Blue is the antidote to red, and it is the primary healing color. Blue is calming, soothing, cooling. Sitting under blue light will help you overcome (or prevent) anxiety and ulcers. It will take away a fever. But don't stay under blue light for more than 30 minutes or you may feel withdrawn and depressed.

If you are "feeling blue," if your energy is depressed, lacking in vitality, if you have a deficiency of passion (red) and need some energy to cheer you up, you might enjoy some red light. You might even drink some red wine and go to the red-light district! If you are a lady and you want some action, get out those red high heels and strut your stuff.

But don't get too carried away, and don't let anger build up inside you for too long, or you are likely to see red, and then there will be no stopping you.

There are many ways to bring color into your life. You can absorb it as colored light; you can apply it to injured bone or tissues in the form of a handheld laser; you can wear it as colored clothing or jewelry; you can ingest it as food, juice, or colored water; you can take it in through your eyes; or you can visualize it through inner vision.

## Antidotes

An antidote counteracts the effect of a substance, as hot antidotes cold and cold antidotes hot. The colors and characteristics of the three lower chakras can be antidoted by those of the three upper chakras, and vice versa. The center (heart) chakra needs no antidote because it has both green and pink. Green is for protection and pink is for vulnerability. So if the heart is overprotected, pink is useful. If the heart feels too vulnerable, green can be comforting.

The concept of antidotes is most useful in dealing with red and blue conditions. When the first chakra has excessive energy, it manifests in conditions that we associate (literally or figuratively) with red, such as inflammation, irritation, body heat, anger, jealousy, and rage. Blue (the color associated with the throat chakra, the first of the three chakras above the heart) can be used to calm and cool the energy of the first chakra or any excessive red condition such as a burn or inflammation.

On the other hand, when the fifth chakra (the throat chakra of communication) has excessive energy, it manifests in blue conditions such as withdrawal, chills, numbness, extreme shyness, and lack of communication. Red can be used to stimulate and warm the energy of the fifth chakra or any excessive blue condition such as the sensation of extreme cold.

The concept of antidotes blurs with the orange and yellow rays, as it does with the indigo and violet rays. Indigo and violet are both purple colors that contain elements of red and blue. Indigo has a greater predominance of blue, and violet has a stronger proportion of red. When orange (the color of the second chakra) is excessive, it becomes red-orange. Then indigo or violet (the colors associated with the sixth and seventh chakras) can be used as antidotes. When yellow (the color of the third chakra) is excessive, it can also become red-orange, and it can be calmed with indigo or violet. Indigo is calming (since it is more blue than red), and violet is more stimulating (since it has more red than blue).

When the sixth chakra is overstimulated, orange is a good antidote. In truth, I have never experienced a problem with excessive crown chakra energy, but if it was a problem, yellow would be the antidote.

This concept of antidotes is essential in color healing, as can be seen in this statement from Dr. Laing:

> If a baby's skin is too red, then the baby is overly excited. This condition should be watched closely, because it can become habitual and lead to red conditions such as heart trouble and high blood pressure in later life. If the baby's mother learns to handle it in early life, these patterns can be changed.
>
> Help the baby to relax. To do this, help the mother to relax. Impress upon her that her relaxation is good for the baby. Give her plenty of blue light. Put her under a blue lamp. Have her wear blue clothes. Listen to soothing music. Bring in blue flowers. Create a soothing environment.[2]

## History of Color Healing

Story-images recorded in cave paintings by Australian Aborigines go back more than twenty thousand years. The serpent is always associated with vibration and flowing energy fields. The Rainbow Serpent is portrayed as a spectrum of various colors, frequencies, and powers that look remarkably like the electromagnetic spectrum. The Rainbow Serpent is attracted to menstrual blood. During fertility rituals people paint themselves with red ocher.[3]

According to ancient Egyptian mythology, the art of healing with color was founded by the god Thoth. To the ancient Greeks, he was Hermes Trismegistus, literally "Hermes thrice-greatest," because of his various works on mysticism and magic. In the Hermetic tradition, the ancient Egyptians and Greeks healed with colored minerals, stones, crystals, salves, and dyes and painted their sanctuaries with healing colors. The ancient Greeks used color to restore balance. Colored garments, oils, plasters, ointments, and salves were employed to treat disease.

In Rome of the first century c.e., Aurelius Cornelius Celsus followed the doctrines established by Pythagoras and Hippocrates, and included the use of colored ointments, plasters, and flowers in several treatises on medicine.

Avicenna (980–circa 1037) was an Arab physician and disciple of Aristotle. In his *Canon of Medicine* he spoke about the vital importance of color in both diagnosis and treatment. He developed a chart relating color to temperament and the physical body. He taught that red moved the blood, blue or white cooled it, and yellow reduced pain and inflammation. He prescribed potions of red flowers to cure blood disorders, and yellow flowers and morning sunlight to cure disorders of the biliary system.

Avicenna wrote also of the possible dangers of color in treatment, observing that a person with a nosebleed, for example, should not gaze at objects of a brilliant red color or be exposed to red light, whereas blue would soothe the condition and reduce blood flow.

Theophrastus Bombastus von Hohenheim (1493–1541) was a Swiss doctor known as Paracelsus. He was familiar with the secret teachings of the Rosicrucians though he was not believed to be a member of that society. Paracelsus is credited with transforming western medicine by improving pharmacy and encouraging scientific experiments, which earned him the title of the Father of Modern Medicine. He considered light and color essential for good health and used them extensively along with elixirs, charms, talismans, herbs, and minerals.[4]

Augustus Pleasanton studied the effects of color in plants and animals and in 1876 he published *Blue and Sun-lights*, stating that the quality, yield, and size of grapes could be significantly increased if they were grown in greenhouses made with alternating blue and transparent panes of glass. He also claimed to cure certain diseases and to increase fertility and the rate of physical maturation in animals. He used color to alleviate human disease and pain.

In *The Principles of Light and Color*, published in New York in 1878, Edwin Babbit used red as a stimulant for the blood, and yellow and orange as nerve stimulants. He claimed that blue and violet were soothing to all systems and had anti-inflammatory properties. Babbit prescribed red for paralysis, consumption, physical exhaustion, and chronic rheumatism; yellow as a laxative, as an emetic and purgative, and for bronchial difficulties; and blue for inflammatory conditions, sciatica, meningitis, nervous headache, irritability, and sunstroke.[5]

Investigations into the therapeutic use of color were carried out in Europe during the early twentieth century. In Austria, Rudolph Steiner (1861–1925) related color to form, shape, and sound, suggesting that the vibrational quality of colors is amplified by certain forms, and that combinations of colors and shapes have either destructive or regenerative effects on living organisms. In the Waldorf Schools inspired by Steiner's work, classrooms are painted and textured to correspond to the moods of children at various stages of their development.[6]

## Color and Light Techniques and Equipment

Dinshah P. Ghadiali (1873–1966) was born in India, and in 1917 he became a United States citizen. He studied chemistry, physics, and electricity in addition to his spiritual practices. In 1891 he was initiated as a fellow in the Theosophical Society.

He developed a method called the Spectro-Chrome System that uses "tonation," treatments with just one color on a given area (or areas), directly on the flesh, for one hour. He used five color filters of red, yellow, green, blue, and violet, and then combined them to obtain the following colors:

Red and yellow = orange
Yellow and green = lemon
Green and blue = turquoise
Blue and violet = indigo
Violet and yellow = purple
Red and violet = magenta
Red and blue = scarlet[7]

Initially he used five glass slides, screening them carefully because each filter had to be a polychrome of suitable proportions to generate appropriate colors when they were mixed. They had to be broad spectrum filters with a preponderance of the primary color. They are called filters because their purpose is to remove (filter out) specific parts from the complete spectrum of white light.

After Ghadiali's death, his son, Darius Dinshah, changed his name to reflect his father's more famous first name, and carried on his father's work by writing *Let There Be Light*. In his book he explains that the intensity of the light source does not make a difference in results. Sunlight may be used by placing large filters over a window, but this can be done only when the sun is shining at a particular angle. A skylight is not acceptable. A treatment can be done outdoors, just by exposing the area, and covering it with the appropriate filters. He recommends closing the eyes during a treatment unless the treatment is intended for the eyes. (This is in direct contradiction to the Syntonics method. Personally, I like to look into the colored light for brief periods.)

Another primitive method is to work indoors, place the filter over the desired area, and shine a flashlight on the area, or tape filters over the head of a flashlight. He emphasizes that *anything* can be used, and gives many examples in his book.

If you want to pursue the therapeutic usage of color healing, Dinshash's *Let There Be Light* is an invaluable resource. It catalogues 331 color schedules with specific tonations for more than four hundred health conditions.

This was the method used by Dr. Kate W. Baldwin (1855–1935), senior surgeon at Philadelphia Woman's Hospital, during the last three of her twenty-three years at the hospital. The following is taken from an abstract of a paper she presented at a clinical meeting of the section on eye, ear, nose, and throat diseases of the Medical Society of the State of Pennsylvania, and published in the *Atlantic Medical Journal* of April 1927.

> Each element gives off a characteristic color wave. The prevailing color wave of hydrogen is red, and that of oxygen is blue, and each element in turn gives off its own special color waves.
>
> If one requires a dose of castor oil, he does not go to a drugstore and request a little portion from each bottle on the shelves. I see no virtue, then, in the use of the whole white light as a therapeutic measure when the different colors can give what is required without taxing the body to rid itself of that for which it has no use, and which may do more or less harm. If the body is sick, it should be restored with the least possible effort. There is no more accurate or easier way than by giving the color representing the lacking elements, and the body will... appropriate them and so restore the normal balance. Color is the simplest and most accurate therapeutic measure yet developed.
>
> For about six years I have given close attention to the action of colors in restoring the body functions, and I am perfectly honest in saying that, after nearly thirty-seven years of active hospital and private practice in medicine and surgery, I can produce quicker and more accurate results with colors than with any or all other methods combined—and with less strain on the patient.[8]

A contemporary physician in Ohio, Teresa E. Quinlin, reports similar results and is equally enthused about the Spectro-Chrome method. "My experience with the lamp is nothing short of stupendous. Burns, infections, pain, and cancer have all had remarkable improvements and successes. A case of the West Nile virus turned around in 72 hours using the color lamp, acupuncture, essential oils, reflexology and the blood type diet. Migraines and fibromyalgia, if not cured, are lessened dramatically. Three cases of ulcerative colitis and/or Crohn's disease are in remission (biopsy proven in two cases). The list goes on."[9]

**Light Box.** A light box should be large enough to accommodate a floodlight or lightbulb. The bottom is constructed so that different colored plates of glass can be inserted and removed.

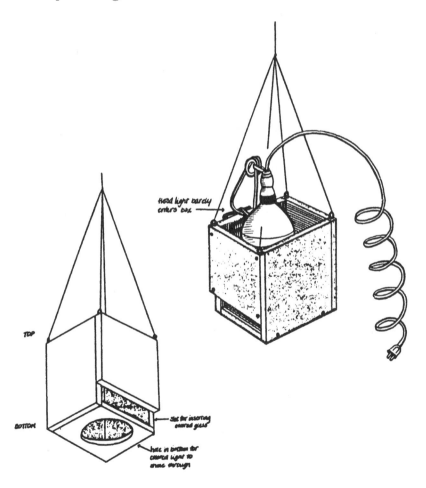

The box that is shown has three side boards, each eight by eleven inches. The fourth side, where the glass or plastic filters slide in and out at the bottom, is eight by nine inches. There is no board at the top; this is where the flood lamp is inserted and clamps in. The bottom board is six by eight inches with a five-inch-diameter round hole that supports the glass and allows the light to shine through. The box is made of hardwood so it is less susceptible to heat and does not become a potential fire hazard if the light is left on and the floodlight is too close to the side. The wood is three-fourths inch thick; this is not necessary, though it gives a firm surface for clamping the light and hanging the chain. The box hangs from a chain, which allows the height to be adjusted, and the chain is fireproof. I'm sure this model can be improved upon.

The goal of color healing is to strengthen and purify each color in your aura. I believe that high-quality German glass gives the purest color and the highest vibratory intensity. In my experience, other kinds of glass are less monochromatic and less effective. Glass or strong plastic is needed if you want to put crystals inside your lamp. Glass can be obtained at stores that sell stained glass.

The lamp may be hung from the ceiling so the light will shine through the glass onto the person seated or lying below. Hang the box so the bottom is six to twelve inches above the part of the body that you are treating.

**Colored Lamp.** A wire frame may be constructed around a lightbulb or floodlight, along with a clamp that holds a plastic gel, so the light shines through the plastic. The whole fixture can be clamped in a suitable place that allows light to shine on the appropriate part of the body. (See Resources.)

**Colored Light Bulb.** Ordinary incandescent lightbulbs are available in red, yellow, pink, green, and blue. They can be inserted into a regular lamp or light fixture. At night or in a darkened room, they will give off a good dose of colored light. Even Christmas lights may be used.

**Stained Glass.** Leonardo da Vinci wrote, "The power of meditation can be ten times greater under violet light falling through the stained glass window of a quiet church." The power of colored light was understood long ago, and may account for the popularity of stained glass windows in churches.

**Colorpuncture.** This technique is described in Peter Mandel's book *Practical Compendium of Colorpuncture*. Mandel employs three sets of opposite colors, comparable to the Chinese yin-yang opposites, to determine the nature of an illness and its treatment. He uses the meridian system and many acupuncture points, but instead of needles, he uses the gentle impulses resulting from light in concentrated form in a kind of flashlight with a pyramid focus tip. He claims that this light spreads out in a fanlike form from the body surface to the tissue below. If a patient experiences discomfort with a particular color, he replaces it with its complementary one. Discomfort indicates an excess of the color and its corresponding vibration in the body.

**Syntonics.** This form of light therapy is used by Dr. Jacob Liberman, based on the work of Dr. Harry Riley Spitler. It works on the concept that most dysfunction is caused by an imbalance between the sympathetic and parasympathetic portions of the nervous system. Filters are divided into three categories: one kind stimulates the sympathetic nervous system, another stimulates the parasympathetic nervous system, a third acts as a physiological or emotional equilibrator.

The practitioner chooses the appropriate color and sets the color dial. The client looks into the box. The color can be arranged to either glow steadily or flash at a designated tempo. As an optometrist, Liberman used Syntonics to treat a vast array of vision problems and vision-related learning problems.

Then he devised his own technique for treating addictions and emotional problems. He would call out pairs of colors (red and blue, yellow and violet, lime and turquoise) and ask the patient to select the set she felt most comfortable with. If she chose red and blue, but preferred blue to red, then red was probably the color she needed for deep healing. The colors that were most disturbing to the patient seemed to represent painful experiences in her life.

At this point I noticed that the behavior of patients with addictive personalities becomes more addictive or less addictive depending on the colors at which they looked. For example, an alcoholic would look at one of the colors to which he was receptive (comfortable with) and be fine; a color to which he was slightly unreceptive might elicit an urge for him to drink juice or soda; a color with which he was most uncomfortable would cause him to want to drink alcohol. It was now becoming clear to me that when situations in life trigger fear or discomfort, our inability to be present with these feelings as well as to deal with them forces us to protect ourselves by avoiding, or *numbing out*, the situations and going into an addictive behavior pattern. . . .

Since the degree of receptivity varied from color to color for each patient, I eventually decided to arrange the colors for treatment from least unreceptive (least uncomfortable) to most unreceptive (most uncomfortable). Starting the treatment with a color that was only mildly uncomfortable allowed patients to gradually develop an authentic security in their ability to go through this process. This would then transfer to their ability to handle stressful situations in their lives. . . .

Although the technology of phototherapy is, in itself, very powerful, its true power blossoms only when the awarenesses that it stimulates can be expressed in the presence of a loving, compassionate human being. In other words, the interaction between the patient and the facilitator is primary. . . .

One of my most important clinical discoveries was that the colors to which people were unreceptive correlated almost 100% of the time with the portions of their bodies [according to the rainbow system of the chakras] where they housed stress, developed disease, or had injured themselves. For example, a person might be uncomfortable looking at the color blue, and during the case history I would discover that this person had chronic sore throats, significant dental problems, [and] difficulty with verbal expression. . . .

Additionally, I noticed that once patients had resolved the emotionally painful issues triggered by the colors, then looking at these colors, which were originally uncomfortable, actually stimulated feelings of joy and euphoria.[10]

**Low Level Laser Therapy.** This therapy is now being used for healing by doctors, dentists, veterinarians, acupuncturists, and laypeople. In Europe it is used for treatment of traumatic, inflammatory, and overuse injuries, pain and healing of arthritic lesions, reduction of abscesses, and treatment of persistent nonhealing wounds such as cold-sores and ulcers. Healing with light and use of low level laser therapy can encourage the formation of collagen and cartilage in damaged joints and the repair of tendons and ligaments.

Infrared light is emitted through some handheld portable low level lasers and other instruments. It has been shown to speed up bone repair by stimulating fibroblastic and osteoblastic proliferation.[11] Cell membranes become more permeable, ATP levels increase, DNA production goes up, and overall cell metabolism becomes more efficient. This seems to be highly stimulating to the cells because they respond rapidly with an increase in density of the capillary bed, reduction of pain and inflammation, stimulation of nerve regeneration, muscle relaxation, and increased muscle tone. There is also an indication that laser light therapy helps increase immune system response.[12]

In addition, low level laser therapy can be used to reduce inflammation and pain by stimulating the release of anti-inflammatory enzymes and endorphins that are natural pain-killing chemicals. It enhances lymphatic draining and releases tight muscles that create chronic pain, joint problems, and decreased mobility. When applied in the correct frequency, low level laser therapy appears to be antiviral, antifungal, and antiherpetic.[13]

Lasers that were once so cost prohibitive that only hospitals could afford them are now in the range of a midpriced computer. Soon I expect that no health professional will be without one, and they will be as common as computers in our homes. (See Lasers page 74 and Resources.)

## Visualization and Color Breathing

For this visualization, close your eyes and picture a color. If it is difficult for you to see yellow, imagine a lemon. Color visualization is most effective when combined with color breathing, as described below.

The colors of the first three chakras, going from bottom to top, are red, orange, and yellow. These are associated with the earth. Visualize these colors arcing up from the earth like half rainbows and entering each of the corresponding chakras. The heart chakra at your chest has two colors: pink and green. Think of one or both of these colors coming directly across the horizon, toward your heart. The top three colors (blue, indigo, and violet) are associated with the heavens. Visualize each of these colors arcing down from the heavens like inverted half rainbows, entering each corresponding chakra.

Imagine you want to bring yellow to your third chakra. Begin by getting a clear mental picture of something yellow. Perhaps you can imagine a lemon. Inhale through your nose and visualize a band of this color arcing up from the earth and flowing into your solar plexus (below your breastbone). As you exhale through your mouth, fix it there.

If you want to send that color to someone else, begin by breathing in the color a few times and fixing it at your own chakra. When you feel that you have enough for yourself, you can send it. The third and sixth chakras are power centers, so they are good transmitting stations. The lower three colors may be sent through the third chakra at the solar plexus, pink and green are sent directly from the heart, and the top three colors may be sent through the third eye.

For example, if you are sending orange, inhale and bring the color to your second chakra (which is orange). Exhale and fix it there. Repeat this several times until you feel you have enough orange. When you are ready to send the color, inhale and bring the orange to the surface of your second chakra, and then bring it up to your solar plexus (without trying to absorb it), and then as you exhale, direct it like a beam of orange light to the person who needs the color. Send it from your solar plexus to the appropriate part of the person's body.

As you exhale, you can also tone, which gives additional vibratory energy. (See Toning for the Chakras, page 171.) Repeat this process three times, then ask the person how it feels. If the results are good, continue until she feels she has had enough (usually six to twelve times). If there is no significant response after six times, it probably is not the color she needs. If she actually feels worse, send the antidote, which, for the second chakra, would be indigo or violet.

Color visualization can be done in the presence of the person you are sending it to or at a distance. The same technique can be used, but instead of directing the color to a person who is directly in front of you, visualize him in your mind and direct the color to that visual image or to a photograph or drawing of him. You may want to focus the color at a particular area of his body. This is remarkably effective, because color healing is energy healing, and energy does not require a person's physical presence. You would not be able to receive verbal feedback about the treatment, so just trust your intuition.

When you send color healing (or any form of energy) to another person, it is best to get his permission first. Not everyone wants to be healed, or even to feel good. However, if a person is unconscious, or unable to speak, or too young to communicate, you can begin by mentally asking permission. Then, unless you feel a definite resistance, you can send healing energy.

One exception pertains to using pink light for self-defense. Pink light is extremely potent. Pink is the energy of love, and when you send pink light in earnest, you must be able to forgive the person you are sending it to. If a person is belligerent, irrational, or irritable, sending pink light is a powerful form of self-defense. It is literally disarming. As soon as she feels the ray of love and forgiveness, she is likely to change her behavior. This may be an invasion of her privacy, but other forms of self-defense would be far more invasive. Here is one example.

One of my students was working at a health food store, and a fellow came in who had had too much to drink. He was being generally obnoxious, insulting the customers and knocking boxes off the shelves. When she asked the man to leave, he ignored her. She was about to call the police when she remembered the pink light. Despite his behavior, she was able to feel compassion as she sent him a strong wave of pink light directly from her heart to his. Within a minute, the man picked up the boxes, apologized for his behavior, and walked out of the store.

(To obtain my cassette tape, *Toning the Chakras*, see Resources.)

## Color-Charged Water

Water can be charged with a particular color and then taken internally or externally. For example, the color of the second chakra is orange, and this chakra is in the area of the large intestines. If there is constipation, it is beneficial to take a few sips of orange-colored water (ambero) before each meal.

When I first heard about color-charged water, I found it hard to believe. The water doesn't look any different after it has been charged. But I am open-minded, and when I got constipated, I decided to give it a try. I could not believe that a few sips would make any difference, so I drank about half a glass before each meal. By evening, I had diarrhea! Since then, I have taken color-charged water more seriously, and it has proven effective for many ailments.

To charge the water, pour into a colored bottle or jar (for example, a green wine bottle or a blue water bottle) and set it on a windowsill so that the light will shine through the glass and into the water. (I would advise against charging all of your drinking water in a blue bottle unless you want to slow down your digestion or unless you have ulcers.) Alternately, you can put a plate of colored glass or a plastic filter against the window and set the water in a clear glass jar or bottle in front of the color source. Or cover the jar with a thin piece of colored cloth. Allow it to stand for one to four hours (four hours may be stronger), and then refrigerate. Take a few sips two or three times a day, as needed.

In cool weather or when refrigerated, red-, orange-, and yellow-charged water will last two to three weeks. In warm weather without refrigeration, it will lose its charge after three or four days.

The other colors will last indefinitely. In fact, green, blue, or purple jars will help preserve oils, herbs, and so on.

The French word for *water* is *eau*, pronounced "o." The following French names are used for colored waters.

Red—*rubio*
Orange and yellow—*ambero*
Green—*verdio*
Blue—*ceruleo*
Indigo and violet—*purpuro*

## Color Healing for the Face

The face is a microcosm of the body, and Dr. Laing explains that the same colors used to treat the chakras can be used to treat the seven areas of the face that correspond to the seven chakras.

1. Red—chin, jaw, lips
2. Orange—inside of mouth, gums, tongue
3. Yellow—throat, leading into intestinal tract
4. Green—nose, leading into respiratory tract
5. Blue—eyes, which are windows to the soul
6. Indigo—ears and third eye
7. Violet—crown chakra

Here are some examples of how to apply this information: During their forties most people experience a waning of sexual energy (second chakra). At this time there is often a deterioration of the gums. This can be treated with a tincture made from calendula (also known as pot marigold, an orange flower) or by rinsing the mouth with *ambero* (orange-charged water).

When the eyes are overstrained, which may occur when you work too hard and don't take enough time for sleep and meditation, the fifth chakra suffers. This condition responds well to placing a smooth blue stone over each eye or by allowing blue light to shine upon your closed eyelids for ten minutes.

## How to Use Color in Your Daily Life

Given the opportunity, your mood will affect your choice of clothes. When you understand the power of color, you can consciously alter your mood. For example, you may be feeling somber and withdrawn and attracted to gray or black. But if you want to cheer up, you would be wise to wear orange, yellow, or pink.

Black, however, is the color of mystery, so if you are in a pleasantly mysterious mood, don't hesitate to wear it. Gray is a neutral color; it doesn't commit you to any particular feeling, so if you are feeling withdrawn, it will leave you that way. But if you are feeling good, gray gives you the flexibility to move through different moods and associate with various kinds of people. You can accessorize neutral colors with colorful scarves, belts, and jewelry.

The color of your underwear can have a strong effect. Red or orange underpants can stir up sexual feelings. Light blue underpants can calm sexual feelings and counteract nervous itching. Red or orange undershirts can cause tension in the back and should not be worn when you have back pain.

The color of clothing can also be used to create a particular impression on those who behold it. Deep purple robes are worn by royalty and religious figures to create an impression of power and devotion. By contrast, bright red is often worn to convey the message of sexual availability.

A masseuse can use pink, green, or yellow sheets on the massage table to encourage clients to breathe deeply (all of these colors strengthen the lungs and diaphragm). In bed, an erotic atmosphere can be created with orange or red sheets and blankets. A cheerful atmosphere can be enhanced with yellow. But a nervous or hyperactive child should never sleep with red, orange, or yellow. A calming green or blue is most desirable.

An argumentative family changed wall-to-wall carpeting from orange to blue, and members got along better afterward. Operatic composer Richard Wagner composed uplifting spiritual music in a room with violet curtains. The color of a room or of furniture influences your mood and health. Yellow cupboards in a kitchen create a cheery atmosphere that is also good for digestion.

Colorful decorations and paintings on the walls will raise the spirits. You can change them when your mood changes.

**Color in Nature.** Nature is full of color, and you can take advantage of her beauty. The way you landscape your home and whether you live near trees, parks, or water can have a profound effect on your well-being. Nature gives a perfect balance of colors, allowing you to choose your favorite colors from her vast array. Be sure to bring in some of your less favorite colors as well, because those are the ones you probably need most. If bright red is distasteful to you, begin with a shade that is less disturbing to you.

I have chosen to live in Hawaii. Seeing large, brilliantly colored flowers all year long—rich reds, outrageous oranges and radiant yellows—feels like a continuous blessing. On clear days, when the sun is bright, the ocean is a brilliant blue. Some days, it is a deep royal blue. Other days it turns emerald green. Sometimes the water close to the coral turns turquoise, while the water farther from shore becomes a rich blue. I inhale those colors and feel as if I am being fed by them.

You may experience being fed by nature if you have been in the city for too long, and you go for a drive in the country and stop to gaze at a meadow of green grass. Breathe in that green and exhale all the dirt and pollution of the city from your lungs. Within a short time, you will feel charged and refreshed. Green feeds the heart chakra, including the lungs. The green of the trees and plants fills the air with oxygen, and those same trees and plants absorb the carbon dioxide that you exhale.

If you are feeling tense after a hard day's work, sit in a comfortable chair outdoors, put up your feet, look at the sky, and soak up that expanse of blue. It is truly remarkable that *wherever* you live on this planet—even in the depths of big cities—the blue of the sky is usually available to you. You can go for a drive and look at the blue expanse of a lake or ocean. Blue is calming and feeds the higher chakras.

When you feel exhausted, you can lie out in the sun and soak up the yellow rays, which feed the third chakra. When the season is right, a bouquet of bright yellow daffodils will cheer up any room, because yellow is the color of happiness.

People who call themselves Breatharians claim not to need food of any kind. I believe that in ancient times there were Beings of Light who simply fed on the colors of nature. I have experienced this on several occasions with rainbows. The first time occurred when I was on a long trip and I was exhausted after driving all day.

I saw a bright and perfect rainbow and pulled off on the shoulder to admire it. I thought how marvelous it would be if I could just gaze at the yellow in the rainbow and inhale its energy. On an impulse, I tried it. Then I watched with amazement as the yellow—*and only the yellow*—of the rainbow turned exceedingly pale. Feeling recharged, rather mind-boggled, and a bit guilty for possibly diminishing someone else's pretty rainbow, I got back in my car and drove away, fairly convinced that it had been an odd coincidence.

Since then I have had this same experience on several occasions. Sometimes just the color I concentrate on will fade, and sometimes the entire rainbow or section of the rainbow that I'm looking at will fade. It seems that the greater my need, the quicker the colors fade. I don't do this for entertainment, because it is sad to see a rainbow fade, and I don't like to deprive myself or others of the opportunity to witness such a blessed sight. I have done this with one or more people, and others have found that they, too, can derive nourishment from the colors of the rainbow.

The *Book of Guidance* says, "Think of a rich green meadow, and as you draw in your breath, inhale the green of the grasses directly into your heart. In ancient times, people did this constantly and automatically. They looked into the expanse of blue sky, and they drew this color into their spirits. They looked at the yellow of the sun, and they drew this warmth into their place of happiness."[14]

**Color in Food and Drink.** In Asian cuisine, the cook often strives to include the four basic colors. When a meal looks appetizing, it is pleasant to eat and easier to digest. A meal that contains the colors of the first four chakras will usually be nutritionally balanced. For example, a meal with tomatoes, carrots, corn, and steamed greens would be pleasant and nutritious. It is good practice to steam the greens until the color is at its brightest; when the greens darken, flavor and nutrition diminish.

The color of food often indicates which parts of the body it will heal. For example, the first chakra is red and relates to the blood. Most of the blood-cleansing foods that tone the liver and lymph glands, eliminating toxins from the blood, are in the red family: red cabbage, cherries, cranberries, blackberries, and red clover tea.

Yellow foods are good for the liver and gall bladder. A flush made from olive oil and lemon juice is excellent for cleansing these organs. Dandelion root tea strengthens the liver and gall bladder.

PART 4

# Healing with the Voice

THE MYSTICS OF NUMEROUS CULTURES AGREE UPON THE ABSO-
lute power of sound. We begin with sound, we are held together by
sound, and someday we will return to the cosmic Music of the
Spheres.

Sound is the original mystical experience of creation. The Sufi
master Hazrat Inayat Khan, a musician of great renown, comments
on the Bible and other great works:

> We find in the Bible the words, "In the beginning was the Word,
> and the Word was God"; and we also find that the Word is Light,
> and that when that light dawned the whole creation manifested.
> These are not only religious verses; to the mystic or seer the deep-
> est revelation is contained in them. . . .
>
> It teaches that the first sign of life that manifested was the audi-
> ble expression, or sound; that is the Word. When we compare this
> interpretation with the Vedanta philosophy, we find that the two
> are identical. All down the ages the Yogis and seers of India have
> worshipped the Word-God, or Sound-God; and around that idea is
> centered all the mysticism of sound or of utterance. Not alone
> among Hindus, but among the seers of the Semitic races too, the
> great importance of the word was recognized. . . . Sanskrit is now
> a language long dead, but in the meditations of the Indian Yogis, San-
> skrit words are still used because of the power of sound and vibra-
> tion they contain. . . .[1]

In 1986, I was privileged to attend a social dance of Coast Salish Indians. It was delightful to be among young and old, with men

117

and women, gathered in a circle around a big drum, each person keeping a constant rhythm with one stick, chanting familiar songs while everyone, including children and old people, danced the simple and graceful steps passed on for generations.

Knowing the power of unifying the communal heartbeat, and the way song and dance give expression to the emotions and the soul, virtually every culture has made use of song and dance, chant and procession, to carry their voices and spirits to the deity of their choice.

The Shoshone, the Coast Salish Indians, and the Huichol Indians of Mexico believe (or used to believe) that the chokecherries won't come back, the salmon won't run, and the sun won't rise unless they chant their prayers of thanks and perform their seasonal rituals. Modern thinkers tend to look upon such ideas as being superstitious or cut off from reality.

Yet when the last traditional Shoshone, the last Coast Salish Indian, the last Huichol Indian, the last of the great trees, and the last of the ancient oil reserves are wiped from the face of the earth, will it surprise us if the salmon do not return (as has happened already in many places), if the chokecherries do not bloom, if the earth shifts on her axis and (as the Hopi predict) if the moon turns the color of blood?

How shall we prevent—or survive—these catastrophes?

Through song. Through finding the voice within. Because if the ancients of every culture can be trusted, life begins with the Word. Through the breath and the Word, we breathe our thoughts into Life. Through the vibratory power of Word and Song, we enter the matrix of vibration from which all of life emerges.

My indigenous friend Craig Carpenter says, "When we sing, we give thanks. And when we give thanks, then miracles begin to happen."

I know this to be true. My life has become a perpetual giving of thanks, and I am constantly amazed by the coincidences, the synchronicity, and the miracles that constantly unfold upon my path. I hear the same testimony from friends and students who take time to meditate, and to give thanks for the blessings of their lives—with words, song, prayer, and silence.

When we believe that we have no one to thank for our good fortune except ourselves, when we neglect to sing and give thanks for what we have; when we believe we are totally separate individuals living in a meaningless universe that has no connection with the Great Mystery or the cosmos, when we believe our songs have no impact upon the universe, then our lives feel empty, and we forget about miracles.

By changing our thinking, remembering to be grateful for all we have, and giving voice to our inner songs, we have the ability to increase our own magnetism, to influence the earth's magnetism, and to create—to give rise to—miracles. I know it. I have seen it.

The way the Australian Aborigines understand (or understood) reality is that energy ordinarily moves very fast. But when it gets an idea, it slows down. When it slows down considerably, it comes into physical manifestation.

The Word is the bridge between energy and material manifestation. Energy becomes sound, and sound transports us into material reality. The spoken or sung word is the most vibratorily powerful manifestor, which is one reason why radio and television are more powerful than newspapers. Native people understand (or understood) the power of using the voice, especially in song, to create and perpetuate the reality they desire.

I believe that when we continually praise life—give thanks for what we have—the energy around us is enlivened, and we become more potent manifestors.

For most North American Caucasians, song and dance are gone from our lives. Too often life is about money: dead paper scalped off proud trees, and precious metals gutted out of sacred places.

Living on this planet today, we are at a painful and thrilling turning point. We can either turn toward a caring, soulful way of life, discovering our inner personal and communal songs, crying out for guidance and miracles, or we can become apathetic and indifferent.

**Sound Healing** is the therapeutic application of sound frequencies to the body/mind of a person with the intention of creating a state of harmony and health. **Toning** is the use of sustained vocal tones, on the out-breath, without the use of melody, rhythm, or words (toning OM, for example). **Sounding** is making improvised sounds without specific melody, rhythm, or words (though melody, rhythm, and words may emerge spontaneously).

## Cultural and Spiritual Uses of Sound

Physics gives us a clue to understanding the power of sound. Scientists used to think that atoms were the tiniest particles of matter until they found that an atom is composed of infinitesimal bits of particle/waves moving in space. In a helium atom, for example, two electrons are held together by an invisible but powerful bond despite distances that are greater, proportionally, than the distance between the earth and the sun.

According to the ancient Hindu science of Ayurvedic medicine, primordial sound is the mysterious link that holds the universe together in a web that is the quantum field. The body is held together by sound, and the presence of disease indicates that some sounds have gone out of tune.[2]

The concept of a web of primordial sound is not unique to Ayurveda. *The Book of the Hopi* by Frank Waters tells of Four Worlds. In the beginning was the Creator, and there was Endless Space. He created Sotuknang, who created solid substance and the waters and air currents. When it was time to create life, Sotuknang created "her who was to remain on that earth and be his helper. . . Spider Woman." He told her, "We see no joyful movement. We hear no joyful sound. What is life without sound and movement?"

Spider Woman took some earth, mixed it with the liquid from her mouth, covered it with a cape made of white substance that was the creative wisdom itself, and sang the Creation Song over it and twins were created. One was to put his hands upon the earth and solidify it to keep it in order. The other was to "send out sound so that it may be heard throughout all the land. When this is heard you will also be known as 'Echo,' for all sound echoes the Creator."

Then, "all the vibratory centers along the earth's axis from pole to pole resounded his call; the whole earth trembled; the universe quivered in tune. Thus he made the whole world an instrument of sound, and sound an instrument for carrying messages, resounding praise to the Creator of all."[3]

The Creator Spirit of the Lakota has no name, and his form is continuously changing, but he is known as Inktomi, the Spider, who is also the Trickster.[4]

The invisible wave patterns that surround us resemble a spider web. I can almost see Spider Woman trapping an idea in her web and weaving it into manifestation. In the ancient Aramaic language of the Bible, the word for prayer translates literally "to set a trap."

In the Hawaiian language the word for song, chant, poem, and prayer is *mele*. A person who composes poetry and chants is *haku mele*. *Haku* is the sorting out of feathers and their arrangement in patterns such as those seen in feather cloaks.

One of the oldest rituals known to the Lakota Indians is the Vision Quest. A person goes into isolation in the wilds, usually on a mountaintop that is considered sacred. The supplicant may be naked, or have the minimal clothing, perhaps a blanket, and no food or water. The ritual is preceded by several days of purification: avoiding sexual intercourse, alcohol, and foul language. There also may be bathing, fasting, taking an enema, and participating in a sweat lodge.

The Lakota word for "to pray" is *cekiya*, derived from *ceya*, "to cry, to lament," with the inserted preposition *ki* meaning "for." From an Indian perspective, prayer and a kind of toning are one and the same, as though you could not speak to the Great Spirit in a normal tone of voice, but must sing, cry, tone, wail, or speak in the ancient sacred language in order to make yourself heard.[5]

Another great Lakota ritual came to Horn Chips in the form of a vision during a Vision Quest he made when he was a young boy. Yuwipi is a Lakota healing ritual. Yuwipi Man is a combination high priest, medium, and shamanic healer to whom the spirits speak during the ceremony, and he brings their messages to the people.

The English word for a Yuwipi gathering is "meeting," but the Lakota word, *lowanpi*, translates as "sing," because there is a lot of singing in this ritual. The leader receives his own songs from the spirits, and he teaches them to the other singers who must be present at every meeting. The songs are repetitious, with just a few lines to each chant, so everyone who attends the meeting is encouraged to join in and "help out." The singers sometimes chant in a whining, high falsetto, or they may sing in a yelping fashion, accompanied by loud drumming. Miraculous healings often occur during these meetings.[6]

The Sun Dance is another powerful ritual of the Lakota that came to a holy man named Kablaya, during a Vision Quest. As instructed, he gathered all the neighboring tribes to participate in the ritual. He taught songs to the singers and told them to bring a large round drum. The ceremony begins with singing and dancing just as the sun comes over the horizon. The singers must sing all day without respite, to hold the tension for the dancers.

In the old days, a sharpened stick was pierced through the dancer's chest, then a leather thong was fastened to the stick and attached to a cottonwood tree that had been brought to the center of the arena. The dancers would lean back on their thongs and dance in the hot sun, all day, without food or water, until the thongs tore open their flesh. Just before sundown a pipe would be brought to the singers and drummers so they could stop and smoke. Later there would be a feast and much rejoicing, for the people felt that a great thing had been done, and the Lakota Nation would be strengthened by this ceremony.[7] The Sun Dance is still performed today, without the piercing.

The Sun Dancers' piercing of the flesh is not unlike the circumcision ceremony that has been practiced by Australian Aborigines for more than 100,000 years. I had the privilege of spending time at an aborigine settlement near Alice Springs a couple years ago, and I believe that some version of this ritual is still being observed. The following is a description drawn from Robert Lawlor's *Voices of the First Day*. When I originally read this book I thought he was describing *all* Australian Aborigines. Now I realize that there are as many different groups of Aborigines as there are different groups of American Indians; each have their own rituals.

This was the ritual that Lawlor observed or heard about from one group.

Several boys are taken into the jungle and decorated with blood from the veins of the older men, to symbolize a new birth in consciousness. They are deprived of food and not allowed to speak while they are kept awake all night for several nights, constantly in the presence of repetitious singing and dancing, until they enter into a trance. Then the older men instruct them, through chanting and singing, about the ancient laws and truths and legends.

Boys are carried like corpses back to the camp, where the wailing women act out their roles as they mourn for the loss of their babies. The women feed the boys, and then the boys are taken on a ceremonial journey away from the village where they join with distant kin of other camps. Later they will return to the original camp for the final ritual.

When they return, the entire village greets them. The women cry and wail, and painted dancers dance around blazing fires until the moment of climax. At this time a group of men rush toward the fire and bend over to form a human table on which the boy is laid. One of his relatives performs the cut with a sharp quartz tool while the grandfather reassures the boy.

Meanwhile the whole community rises to a frenzy of dancing, singing and moaning while whirling the humming bullroarers (wooden rods with lashes that, when twirled, produce a low humming sound). The cutting ceremony is a test of the boys' ability to enter into a trance state where they will not feel pain.

When the circumcision is complete, the boys remain in seclusion, where they are not allowed to speak, except by sign language. The all-night dance ceremonies continue while the old men instruct the boys about their sacred responsibility toward the earth and the nature of the journey they must make after death.

Immediately after the circumcision, each young man is presented with two bullroarers and told that they are his new parents, and he should call on them when he is in need. The bullroarers hold the hypnotic power that gives him entry into the Dreamtime.[8]

It is uncanny how similar certain aspects of the Aborginal circumcision ceremony is to the "grabbing" of reluctant candidates for the Spirit Dance of the Nooksack Coast Salish Indians of northwestern Washington. During this dance participants become possessed by a song, *syowen*, that comes and demands to be expressed.

A person is most likely to have this experience while he or she is in a highly susceptible condition: during a fever, or while grieving over the death or loss of a loved one, or even during times of extreme anger toward a loved one. The person might weep continually until her cries turn into the characteristic groans of a Spirit Dancer. Then it is said that the *syowen* takes pity on the unhappy person.

Alternately, if a loved one is stricken by cancer or some other dread disease, a person can become a Spirit Dancer to help heal her beloved. Spirit Dancers are believed to have protection from sickness as well as accidents, and usually live to a ripe old age.[9]

In the late 1970s, about 20 percent of the Coast Salish participated in this ceremony (I don't have more current information). "Grabbing" was the most popular way of getting new members. A family might set up a youth to be grabbed because of a drinking problem, or difficult and rebellious behavior. The boy or girl had to be at least semi-willing to be grabbed, and the family had to be fully willing because of all the ritual obligations it entailed.

Like practices of Australian Aborigines, when a candidate is chosen, a number of men from the dancing community literally grab the young person, lift him up, and carry him away, keeping him awake and isolated for a prolonged period in a condition of sensory deprivation, combined with singing and drumming, until the weary candidate falls into a trance when he tends to have visions, usually of an animal spirit helper. The person's power, song, and dance come from this helper.

When the person is seized by the dance and song family and friends gather to sing and drum, pouring their own feelings into the singing of the song. The dancer experiences release and fulfillment. "When the drumming is right, it feels like floating!"[10]

The Pentecostal Church is one of many religions adopted by Native Americans. It is popular among the Coast Salish, because it so nearly resembles their own trance experiences. At Pentecostal and Baptist Churches, possession is condoned when it is expressed through *speaking in tongues*, which is very similar to the *syowen* possession.

Here is a description of the experience by a woman who was a member of the Pentecostal Church as a child in Southern California:

> After the sermon, the Minister would pray for the sinners and give them a chance to come down and be saved—to submit themselves to Christ. The whole church would be in a meditation-type place where they'd all be praying. I'd close my eyes, and the prayer would seem to go on forever. I could hear through the church that people were more or less talking under their breath and saying things like "Dear Jesus!" and giving praise to God, and telling Him how good He is, and thankful and hallelujah.
>
> And if you felt called then you could walk down the aisle to the front, to the altar and get down on your knees and let everybody witness the fact that you are giving your heart to Jesus. And there might be other people up there at the same time. So while you're down on your knees praying for your sins, of course you're crying; it gets very very emotional. All the things you've done wrong are coming up and out.
>
> And when you do that, the church leaders will come down and lay their hands on you and pray for you. And it just seems that the energy is so great; it's just an incredible feeling. I remember when I did that and we had a visiting minister and he laid hands on me and I went under the power of the Holy Ghost. I fell totally backwards, almost in a faint. I guess people helped me down, because I just went backwards and I was just layin' there mumbling. And then I just came up with this verbiage that I could hear in one realm, but in the other, I wasn't a part of it. I just didn't have control over my tongue.
>
> So that's when you're making all the sounds, and talking in tongues. It never really sounded like another language. I can't even do it. I can't mimic it. There were a lot of rolls, a lot of la-la-la-la. But you do repetitively use the same syllables again and again to

get into the power of it. It has a certain lilt to it. It's a song without a lot of ups and downs.

When it's over, it just naturally goes into "Oh Jesus, thank you God." You do feel like you've been close to God. And once you do that, there is a complete lightening up of your burdens. It feels like you have no cares, because now they are in God's hands. Then thereafter, when you pray after church services, it just comes out again.[11]

All of these rituals are true spiritual experiences in which the participants actually touch the spirit realms with the assistance of toning, chanting, and singing. They are not empty rituals, nor are they likely to be works of magic or trickery. The results may be miraculous healings, but the deeper purpose is expressed in the most beloved song of the Sun Dancers:

Wakantanka pity me.
I want to live; that's why I am doing this.[12]

**Seed Sounds.** Certain tones, including vowel sounds, have been used in ancient cultures throughout the world to increase and decrease energies before they manifest on the material plane. The Australian Aborigine hunters knew that certain rhythms and sounds coagulate (increase) or disperse (decrease) the premanifesting energies of each species. They believed that the earth's magnetism or Rainbow Serpent (not unlike our electromagnetic spectrum) creates the creatures of this plane. According to Lawlor, before going hunting for a particular animal, the hunters would make the designated Seed Sounds "at the place where the potency of that creature was deposited in the Dreamtime" in order to increase that animal's fertility and abundance.[13]

Perhaps this is not so far-fetched. The seed of the body is in the genitals. Human increase and decrease in population depends upon the fertility or sterility of our seeds. Music and song almost always accompany dance, certain music and dancing may be regarded as a kind of foreplay, and music often accompanies sexual expression.

In the Celtic tradition, Beltane, the last of three spring fertility festivals, occurs on May 1st and is often accompanied by a Maypole Dance. Few people realize that "the maypole is a frank symbol of the male principle, while the flower crown represents the womb. The maypole channels the Earth's energy through the circlet around its top, bringing fertility to all who dance around it. . . . For the villagers, it was a festival of unashamed sexuality, as couples made love freely in the fields and gardens to bring fruitfulness to the crops."[14]

The Hindus also have seed sounds. They call them *bija*, and they believe certain vibrations manifest as sounds corresponding to the different color vibrations of each chakra. Each chakra is seen as a kind of lotus with a designated number of petals, and each of the petals has a sound. Thus all fifty sounds within the Sanskrit language are contained within the chakras. Harish Johari, a North Indian musician, composer, poet, artist, and Tantric scholar, produced a tape of these "Sounds of the Chakras"[15] (see Resources).

**Healing Broken Bones.** I have come across two entirely separate accounts of almost instantaneous healings of broken bones from two separate cultures, both of which involve sound.

Max Freedom Long in *The Secret Science Behind Miracles*, originally written in 1948, recounts the story of his good friend, J. A. K. Combs of Honolulu, a fellow student of Hawaiian *kahuna* teachings. Combs's grandmother-in-law was one of the most powerful *kahuna* or healers on the island of Oahu.

Combs was invited to a beach party at the country home of the elderly kahuna. Combs watched as one Hawaiian guest arrived at the party, slightly intoxicated. The man missed his step from the car to the soft sand and fell. As he fell, there was the characteristic snapping sound of breaking bones. Inspection showed two bones protruding through the skin above the ankle. Combs, who had himself suffered such a compound fracture, prepared to take the man to the hospital.

Instead the elderly kahuna arrived. She straightened the leg and gently placed the bones together, pressing on the area where the ends of the bone pushed out through the skin as she began a low chanted prayer. In a short time she fell silent. Her hands suddenly moved, and she took them away from his leg and said softly in Hawaiian, "The healing is finished. Stand up. You can walk." The injured man, now completely sober, stood and took one step in amazement, then another. The healing was complete and perfect, and the leg showed no sign of a break.[16]

It is remarkable how similar this description is to Marlo Morgan's account, in *Mutant Message Down Under*, of an event she says she witnessed while traveling with a group of Australian Aborigines. According to Morgan, one of the male hunters was walking at the edge of an embankment when the ground gave way and he plunged down twenty feet. His companions hoisted him up to the top and set him on a slab of rock; he had a severe compound fracture between the knee and ankle. "The bone was protruding like a huge ugly tusk, about two inches through the milk chocolate-colored skin," she wrote.

The Aborgines called Medicine Man and Female Healer stood on either side of the injured man. Morgan moved up close and watched as Medicine Man moved his hands up and down the wounded leg about an inch away from the surface in a gentle gliding motion, first parallel and then alternating, with one hand sliding up as the other slid down. The injured man and both healers all began to speak in prayerlike fashion. Medicine Man put both hands around the ankle, and Female Healer kneeled at the man's side and put both hands around the man's knee. They chanted or sang at the same time, though each one's song was different, until they all raised their voices in unison and shouted something. Morgan did not see any pulling. "The bone just slipped back into the hole from which it had exited."

Finally Medicine Man held the ragged skin together and Female Healer used a kind of black tar (made from clots of menstrual blood) to cement the wound together. Morgan wrote: "The next morning, Great Stone Hunter stood up and walked with us. There was not a hint of a limp. The ritual they had performed, they told me, would reduce the osseous stress and prevent swelling. It had worked. For several days I looked closely at his leg and watched as the natural black compound dried and began falling off. Within five days it was gone; there were only thin scarlines where the bone had exited."

How could the body heal so instantaneously? According to Morgan, "I was told that the movement of the hands up and down, over the area of involvement, without touching, was a way of reconnecting the former pattern of the healthy leg. It would eliminate any swelling during the healing phase. Medicine Man was jogging the memory of the bone into acknowledging the true nature of its healthy state. This removed the shock created when it snapped in half, ripping away from the position developed over thirty years. They 'talked' to the bone."[17]

Max Freedom Long asked the kahunas how they could instantly heal a broken bone, and they responded that "the shadowy (*aka*) body of the low self is a mold of every cell of the body, also of its general shape…to heal a broken bone, the High Self dissolved the injured bone and other tissues into ectoplasm, this usually being invisible, but not always. As the shadowy body mold is made of invisible substance, it cannot be broken or injured. Thus, with the mold of the normal leg there at hand, the ectoplasmic material of the dissolved parts is resolidified in the mold, with the result that the healing is instant and the limb is restored to its former condition."[18]

## Author's Experience with Sounding

When I lived near Taos, New Mexico in 1967, my Apache friends invited me to attend a meeting of the Native American Church, to bless their new land. I heard that a Road Man (a holy man who conducts these all-night ceremonies) named Little Joe would be coming from Taos Pueblo, and he wanted to be sure that there would be at least six people who knew the songs so they could hold the energy. Our host reassured him that this would happen.

When I arrived toward evening, the sun was already low on the horizon, painting the mesas in a brilliant salmon-colored wash. A tall, resplendent tepee graced the land. Little Joe arrived with a couple men from the Pueblo who would assist him with the ceremony. He was a diminutive man with a remarkable combination of humility and wisdom.

We gathered outside the tepee—about twenty of us—as the sun went down behind the mesa. Little Joe invited us to come in and we packed inside, just barely fitting around the circumference, cross-legged, with our knees scrunched up against each other. Little Joe sat directly across from the entrance, facing east. Then the Cedar Man came in and closed the flap. He tended the fire.

We were asked not to fall asleep and not to leave the tepee for any reason without asking permission of the Cedar Man, because everyone who began the meeting should be there at the end, at sunrise, to keep the energy together.

Little Joe passed the Bull Durham (pure Virginia tobacco) around the circle, and we each rolled our own ritual cigarette, took a few puffs, and made a prayer. The smoke would carry our prayers to the Great Spirit. We placed our cigarettes on the nearly circular road that Joe drew in the sand in front of us, and the chanting began. Joe murmured some prayers in his own language, and there was more chanting. Joe passed the drum to the man on his right and held onto the rattle. The person who holds the rattle speaks or sings while the person on their right accompanies on the drum.

Little Joe spoke in English and said something like this: "Ho! Heavenly Father, Earthly Mother, thank you for this fire tonight and all these good people who've come to walk this road with us and bless this land. Thank you for this beautiful day and all the women who came to help us cook. Thank you for this good path that you've given us to walk." He shook the rattle and his assistant took up the drum. The group broke into a lively chant.

Little Joe shook the rattle again and continued, "Great Spirit, I want to ask you to watch over my neighbor, Jim, 'cause he had a real bad accident two days ago when he fell off that combine and wrenched his shoulder. His wife is havin' a hard time takin' care of him and the kids, too. HO!" (He shook his rattle for emphasis, and several people said "Ho!" in agreement.)

Joe passed the rattle to George on his left. George was one of the men from the pueblo. The drum was passed to Little Joe, so he could play for George. There was a lot of chanting and then

George said, "Ho, Great Spirit, Father-Mother. We're traveling this road tonight, this good road that you have given to our people. We want to ask you to bless this land and take good care of Jake and Jim and Sandy and Inez, so there will be plenty of water, and the crops will grow tall, and there will be plenty of food to eat.

"I want to ask you to help my mother, because that arthritis is getting pretty bad in her back and it's been hard for her to get out of bed these past few days. She wanted to be here tonight, but she just wasn't strong enough to make the trip. I want to ask you to comfort her and make that back strong again. HO!" The rattle shook while other folks from the pueblo joined in the Ho! I could feel that they all knew his mother and cared about her and were sending her lots of good energy. Then they all broke into a lively chant. The energy was beginning to build.

Around midnight, a woman from outside brought a big pot of medicine tea to the entrance of the teepee. The Cedar Man received it, and passed it around. After we drank the tea, the energy picked up some more, the chanting intensified, and the prayers seemed more impassioned.

Never before had I heard ordinary people talking directly to God! I came from a culture where not even priests or rabbis talked to God. Where I came from, everyone in his or her right mind knew that only crazy people thought they could talk to God. But these people, whose lives had such direct simplicity, were teaching me something different.

As I listened to the drumming, chanting and praying, trying to avoid the smoke of the fire, I could feel my weariness and it was difficult to resist lying down. I found myself almost sleeping in a sitting position, rocking back and forth in rhythm to the repetitive chanting and drumming.

There was something so familiar and comforting about the rocking movement and the deep chanting in a foreign tongue. The word *davenning* came to mind. I felt myself transported to a different place and time. I was a small child, rocking in my mother's lap. We were at the sumptuous synagogue in Chicago during one of the special Holy Days. I'm sure my mother was remembering the High Holy Days during her childhood in Poland, when all the neighbors came flocking to her father's home. She was watching her beloved father, who was both Rabbi and Cantor for their little village, with his great bushy beard and the *yarmulka* perched on his abundant black hair. He was wrapped in his white prayer shawl, praying, *davvening* (rocking back and forth), chanting over the sacred prayer book.

Those early experiences at the Synagogue must have been my first awakening to spirituality. The combination of my mother's devotion and the soulful chanting of the Cantor, in an ancient language, transported me to a deeply profound place. It was like the native chanting in the teepee.

The rattle was being passed to the man on my right, and he was praying aloud. This was the second time it had gone around the circle, and it would be my turn soon. I did not speak the first time. I had no idea what to say. Throughout the night I had been listening to the native people chanting and praying aloud for their friends, their neighbors, their animals, their crops, for the boys in Vietnam, for the President of the United States, and for their parents. Suddenly it felt strange that I had not spoken to my parents in two years; I didn't even know where they were.

When my family moved to California and joined the reform temple, I was shocked that there was no Cantor, no one to chant the Hebrew prayers. I could not feel God in those services. They felt empty, shallow, devoid of spirit and passion. At the age of eight, I refused to go back to that place where women went to show off their fancy new clothes. The temple felt superficial, full of hypocrites pretending to worship God.

So I turned my back on religion, and I became cynical. But I was still searching. Sometimes my Grandfather would come to me in visions. I never met him in the flesh, because he died in a concentration camp in Poland. But he would tell me things about himself, and when I shared these experiences with my mother, she confirmed that what he said to me was true.

As I grew older and left home, I continued my spiritual quest. My parents were critical of the lifestyle of simplicity and poverty that I chose in the 1960s. And I was fiercely judgmental of their conspicuous over-consumption. Eventually my mother disowned me and for two years we did not communicate. Now I had a six-month-old baby and my parents had never seen their grandchild.

During the chanting in the teepee, I had a deep experience of Spirit for the first time since I was a child. As I listened to the Indian people chanting and praying aloud for their parents, my judgments toward my own parents softened.

I must have been nodding out because I was startled when the man on my right began shaking the rattle. Everyone was chanting intently. My body rocked in rhythm to the chanting and suddenly I could hear my grandfather talking. My heart swelled with joy. It had been such a long time!

He showed me an endless line of people—all related—holding hands. My grandfather stood on the far side of my mother, holding her right hand with his left, while his own right hand joined a chain of relatives that seemed to stretch to infinity. My mother's left hand hung limp and useless at her side, while my right hand refused to take hers. I could feel the break of energy between us and the grief it caused my grandfather. I could feel how much effort it took for me to reach him and my other kin as long as that link was broken.

Tears flowed down my cheeks and my heart ached as the rattle was passed to me. I had feigned indifference toward my parents, but now the energy flowed from my heart to my throat as I broke into a wordless chant that seemed like a combination of the High Holy Day songs that I dimly remembered and the Indian chants that I'd been hearing all night. I didn't care what anyone thought; my soul poured out of my mouth as I expressed my grief, my sorrow, and my longing for the connections I did no longer had.

When I was done I shook the rattle fiercely and everyone shouted "HO!"

That was my first experience of sounding, though I didn't even know the word then. Many years would pass before I would dare to open up my voice like that again. But it was the beginning. I connected my heart with my mouth.

When I left Little Joe, I found my parents and mended the link with my mother, bridging that gap so that my children would know their grandparents and all the relations would be connected. As I entered the world outside the teepee, I knew that I had a direct connection with Spirit. I felt it when I was chanting.

## Sound, Science, and Medicine

We do not live in a void. The seemingly empty space around us is full of invisible sound and light waves. We influence that space and are influenced by it. Most of us are unaware of our effect upon it and its effect upon us. Yet we can become intelligent and active participants in this cosmic drama. We can learn to work the miracles that were once reserved for Shamans and esoteric schools of healing.

Sound is the key.

Let us begin in the womb. For eighteen weeks your cells have been growing and multiplying. You can feel, move, and even respond to stimuli.

Then something dramatic happens that changes you forever. Suddenly *you can hear*! The ear is the first organ to develop in embryo.[19]

Here is quote from my own book (currently out of print), *Healing Yourself During Pregnancy.*

> One of my clients told me that there were certain passages from the Bible that he early loved and easily learned by heart. Later his mother told him that those were the passages that she had read aloud, over and over, during her pregnancy with him. . . .
>
> With my first child, I was in labor for thirty-six hours. The last several hours were filled with painful contractions. I had been trained in the Lamaze method, and I made good use of the pant-and-blow technique consisting of three short pants followed by a long blow. For several days after my son was born, he had a peculiar habit of taking three short pants followed by a long blow![20]

John Ortiz, Ph.D., director of the Institute of Applied Psychomusicology, a licensed psychologist in central Pennsylvania, and author of *The Tao of Music*, cites many sources for current research in the effects of music on healing.[21] Music is now making its way into the hospital wards of premature infants. Researchers found that lullabies rapidly cause an increase in oxygen saturation levels as well as heart and respiration rates.[22]

Autistic and developmentally disabled children benefit significantly from the use of music, displaying better pragmatic skills[23] and increased positive participation in social activities with less disruption.[24] They are better able to focus, they show fewer symptoms of boredom,[25] and they have better recall.[26]

While adults tend to have a negative reaction to the driving beat of heavy metal music, it seems to be beneficial for adolescents who are overcome by anger, fear, and feelings of hopelessness.[27]

Adults also benefit from the effects of music. Several studies show an increased ability to tolerate pain.[28] As mentioned elsewhere, Dr. Mitch Gaynor, oncologist, had the same experience with many patients with cancer, and with a woman who had fibromyalgia.[29] Many of my clients have thrown away their pain medications. (See the exercise, Toning for the Pain in Your Body, page 164.) Here is the story of one of my students, Karen McDaniel:

In late 1998 a recurring foot infection took me back to the large university medical center where I had previously received a pancreas/kidney transplant (having had Type I diabetes for 35 years). The third day, an intern announced that the toe next to the big toe on my right foot was completely dead and needed to be amputated immediately.

The surgery went smoothly, and with the prayer support of caring friends I was able to send healing energies to my right foot. The only problem was that the throbbing pain proved unbearable, in both the amputation site and in the "phantom toe." High-powered pain relievers with codeine couldn't touch this pain that kept me edgy and unable to sleep.

I had attended Joy Gardner's Vibrational Healing Intensive a few months previously, and I thought she might be able to help. So I called and she offered to spend five minutes each day for the next couple weeks, toning directly into the toe, over the phone. (She was in Hawaii, and I was in Ohio.)

On our first call, I held the receiver down to my foot and I could feel her tones reaching out to make contact with my toe. Then they changed and the sounds seemed to become the voice of the toe, expressing outrage and distress. This went on for some time. She finished by sending peaceful, healing tones, which soothed and quieted the throbbing pain.

After that session, the pain was less sharp and less insistent. On the following days, she repeated similar toning, and by the third day, the pain was gone by the end of the session. It did return after a few hours, but with less intensity. Each day, the alleviation of pain improved, and the pain-free time increased.

A comical incident occurred one day when Joy was in the midst of a toning session. I was diligently holding the telephone receiver at my foot when along comes the Chief Surgeon making his rounds, followed by his flock of white-coated minions. I insisted on completing my sound treatment and they all stopped in total amazement to hear the sounds pouring out of the phone toward my foot!

After a few days I had enough strength to try some light toning for myself in between Joy's treatments. Luckily I was in a private room.

By the second week, I stopped asking for other pain relievers. When I was back at home, I toned for myself during the rare times when the pain recurred. My body seemed to instruct me when the toning needed to change, and I began doing what felt like a knitting-together tone, going in-and-out, like a needle and thread. In the end, my skin—which was not expected to heal well, due to diabetes and immune-suppressant drugs—healed beautifully.

Musician Jim Oliver concurs that the body is capable of responding to sounds that the ears do not necessarily hear. He put specific sounds into a pair of headphones and set them on a client's ankles with positive results. He believes that the blood cells quickly carry the resonance throughout the whole body.[30]

During the 1990s researchers produced many reports about the tranquilizing effects of music on physical and mental health. But few studies used rigorous methodologies or adequate sample sizes, and results were inconsistent. Also there was disagreement concerning the type of music that should be offered to patients. In 1994 an abstract by Karen Allen and J. Blascovich was reported in the *Journal of the American Medical Association* titled "Effects of Music on Cardiovascular Reactivity Among surgeons." In this study the surgeons' cardiovascular responses to music were calmed as they performed stressful tasks while listening to self-selected music as well as experimenter-selected music. The study concluded that familiarity with and control over selection of music produced positive physiological response, whereas the music that was presumed to be sedative did not produce consistent results.

In a second study from the State University of New York at Buffalo, Karen Allen, a psychologist, and Lawrence Golden, a cardiologist, followed elderly patients undergoing eye surgery at an ambulatory clinic where they would go home on the same day as the surgery. This process was known to be stressful, especially for older patients who were not accustomed to such procedures. Forty patients were selected. Twenty-one had drug-controlled high blood pressure, ten in the experimental group and eleven in the control group. They did not stop using their medications.

One week before surgery, their blood pressure and heart rate were taken as a baseline. At that point there was no significant difference between the two groups. On the day of the procedure, the same vital signs were taken before, during, and after the surgery. Participants in the experimental group were given stereo headphones, a cassette player, and a choice of twenty-two types of music including soft hits, classical guitar, chamber music, folk music, and popular singers from the 1940s and 1950s. No more than three individuals selected the same type of music. Control group participants were left to rest quietly without headphones or music.

Both groups showed significantly higher heart rates and blood pressure at the clinic than the baseline measurements when they arrive. The experimental group was provided with music, and diminished physiological effects occurred within five minutes. During surgery, the patients provided with music had heart rate and blood pressure values similar to the baseline rates taken one week previously. The control group had persistent elevations in blood pressure similar to preoperative levels. Patients with music reported a dramatic reduction of stress and increased coping abilities, whereas those without music did not.

When participants using music were interviewed, they repeatedly mentioned the word *control* noting that when they entered the facility they immediately felt as if they were relinquishing all personal control. Given a choice of music helped restore a small amount of personal control. It also blocked out "the chatter of the doctors and nurses." In the previous study reported in the *JAMA*, surgeons also felt strongly that the ability to control the type of music enhanced their abilities to perform cognitive tasks and influenced reactivity.[31]

A study at Michigan State University in 1993 allowed experimental subjects to select music from one of four categories: New Age, mild jazz, classical, and impressionist. Control subjects were given only magazines. After just fifteen minutes, the experimental group showed an increase in blood levels of interleukin-1 from 12.5 to 14 percent. Interleukins are a family of proteins associated with blood and platelet production and lymphocyte stimulation. They help protect cells against invasion by AIDS, cancer, and other diseases. In this study, participants showed decreased levels of cortisol by as much as 25 percent. Cortisol, a steroid hormone associated with the adrenal complex, is related to stress and susceptibility to inflammatory diseases. The scientists concluded that preferred music "may elicit a profound positive emotional experience that can trigger the release of hormones which can contribute to a lessening of those factors which enhance the disease process."[32]

In 2004 researchers at Ohio State University took thirty-three heart patients who had undergone bypass surgery or angioplassty. These procedures carry a risk of cognitive impairment. The patients were given fluency tests before and after two separate sessions of exercising on a treadmill. During one session they heard Vivaldi's *Four Seasons*. While all the participants felt better after working out on the treadmill, the verbal fluency after listening to the music increased by more than double.[33]

Other studies show that music can be used to alleviate depression, anger, and loneliness, and improve awareness and insight.[34] It can increase motivation, endurance, and psychological well-being and physical comfort, as well as alleviate anxiety and enhance relaxation.[35]

One of my graduate students, Cynthia Mitchell (see Resources), a former theater teacher at Duke University in North Carolina, was hired by the Health Arts Network at Duke Hospital to sing for the patients. She would go into a room, chat with the patients (and their families, if present), and inquire if they had any special song requests. After singing a familiar song or two, she would tune in on the energies of the patient and ask permission to improvise a special song. Using her intuition to sense the sounds needed, Cynthia would watch as the patient's breathing slowed and deepened, her face relaxed, and tension left her body.

One evening, as she was passing an intensive care room, the nurse on duty asked Cynthia if she would come in and sing for her patient. The woman's heart rate had been dangerously high (between 120 and 94) all night. Cynthia came into the room, tuned in on the woman, and knew exactly what sounds to make. When she finished singing, as she turned to leave, the nurse put her hand on Cynthia's shoulder. There was a look of amazement on her face as she whispered, "While you were singing, her heart rate dropped by twenty points!" A few hours later, before leaving for the night, Cynthia stopped by to check on the woman and the nurse told her gratefully that the woman's heart rate had stabilized at 74.

How does sound affect the emotions? One explanation is that when it passes through the ear, it activates the vagus nerve that extends from the ear down into the larynx and through the entire intestinal tract, where its fibers control gastric and pancreatic secretions. This is in the area of the third chakra, which is an emotional center. The vagus nerve also has inhibitory fibers that pass through the heart,[36] which is in the area of the fourth chakra, another emotional center.

In fact, sound is a kind of food for the brain and the body (to say nothing of the soul). Dr. Tomatis, a French physician, psychologist, and auditory neurophysiologist, found that the brain requires three billion stimuli per second for at least four and a half hours per day *just to stay awake!* He claims that the ear produces over 90 percent of the body's total charge.[37]

Surely this explains why so many young people seem to be addicted to music with a driving beat. It literally acts as a stimulant. When you need a shot of energy, music can give it to you. During the 2003 invasion of Iraq, the soldiers in the United States army listened to CDs inside their tanks as they attacked. One popular song selected for the occasion was *"The Roof is on Fire,"* by the Bloodhound Gang, which includes the following verse:

The roof the roof the roof is on fire
The roof the roof the roof is on fire
The roof the roof the roof is on fire
We don't need no water let the motherf——r burn
Burn motherf——r burn .[38]

What better way for young men to overcome their dread of taking human lives than to listen to loud, incessant, aggressive music in an isolated cage that resembles a booth at a video parlor?

Dr. Tomatis claims that the ear is the conductor of the entire nervous system. Through the medulla (the brain stem), the auditory nerve connects with all the muscles of the body. Thus muscle tone, equilibrium, flexibility, and vision are all influenced by sound.[39] This helps explain why, when yoga is accompanied by toning, it becomes possible to stretch longer and deeper. It also explains why most people like to hear music while they exercise.

According to Dr. Tomatis, high frequency sounds (3,000 Hz and above) increase the electrical potential of the brain.[40] The music of Mozart has also been credited with increasing mental powers, as made popular by Don Campbell in his book, *The Mozart Effect*. He cites a study by Frances H. Rauscher, Ph.D., and her colleagues in which thirty-six undergraduates from the psychology department scored eight to nine points higher on a spatial IQ test after listening to ten minutes of Mozart's Sonata for Two Pianos in D Major. The effect only lasted for ten to fifteen minutes, but the team concluded that there was a strong relationship between listening to this music and spatial reasoning.[41]

Don Campbell points out that the right ear relays auditory impulses more quickly to the speech centers in the brain than does the left ear. Nerve impulses from the right ear go directly to the left (rational) brain, where the speech centers are located. However, nerve impulses from the left ear have to make a circuitous journey through the right brain, which is devoid of speech centers, before they end up at the left brain. This results in a subtle loss of attentiveness and ability to respond verbally.

Consequently Campbell advises situating yourself so that a person is slightly to your right while conversing, and holding the telephone to your right ear to improve listening, focus, and retention of information.[42]

Dr. Tomatis became acutely aware of how important the voice is in charging the body when he was called to a Benedictine monastery in France where the monks were well known for sleeping little, eating a simple vegetarian diet, observing silence, and chanting six to eight hours a day. This monastery had just been taken over by a young abbot who was convinced that chant served no useful purpose and had eliminated it. Within a short time, seventy of the ninety monks complained of feeling inexplicably fatigued.

The doctors who were brought in tried prescribing more sleep and adding meat to the diet, but this only made things worse. When Dr. Tomatis arrived, he promptly prescribed a return to their usual schedule of chanting. Within five months, most of the monks returned to their normal health and vigor.[43]

Gregorian chants are a collection of chants taken from various cultures and standardized into the Catholic Mass by St. Gregory (pope from 590 to 604 C.E.). They differ from ordinary music because the timing is not according to meter, but depends upon the ability of the singers to chant on a prolonged exhalation. The training takes four years before a novice is brought into the choir.[44]

Because the chants are based on the breath, they have a powerful effect on the listeners, who soon find themselves taking deep breaths, which in turn slows down their hearts and reduces their blood pressure. Tomatis explains, "If you put an oscilloscope on the sounds of Gregorian chant, you see that they all come within the bandwidth for charging the ear. There is not a single sound which falls outside of this."[45]

Listening to Gregorian chants helps create a state of calm and an increase in energy, memory, and concentration. I often listen when I am writing because it keeps my mind calm and prevents my body from holding tension. Tomatis explains that music in relatively low frequencies (such as shamanic drumming) affects the more primitive areas of the brain, creating a hypnotic state, whereas the Gregorian chants stimulate the cortex, making you feel alert.[46]

A study of thirty-two choir members in Irving, California, in 2001 confirmed the benefits of singing in a choir. They performed Beethoven's choral masterwork, *Missa Solemnis*. Researchers used cotton swabs to collect saliva, which contains the immune protein Immuno-globulin A, used by the immune system to fight disease.

According to the study, the protein increased 150 percent during rehearsals, and by 240 percent during performance. The boost seemed directly related to the singers' states of mind, which many participants described as happy or euphoric. "Afterward, I'm floating," said Morris, age sixty-one, a member of the choir. "I feel terrific. There have been many times going into a concert when I'm fighting a cold or have a sore throat, but I managed to show up and do the performance, and I'm higher than a kite when it's over."

Education professor Robert Beck, who coauthored the study with Thomas Cesario, concluded that, "The more passionate you feel while singing, the greater the effect."[47]

**Resonance and Entrainment.** The principles of resonance and entrainment are basic to understanding how Vibrational Healing works. In 1665 Dutch mathematician Christian Huygens (1629 to 1695) was working on the design of pendulum clocks. He found that when two clocks were mounted on a wall near each other, even though the pendulums were swinging at different rates, they would eventually end up swinging in sync with each other. He discovered that the powerful rhythmic vibrations of one object will cause a less powerful object to lock into the vibration of the dominant source.

Similarly, when individual pulsing heart muscle cells are brought close together, they begin pulsing in sync with each other.[48] In sound healing, the practitioner may begin by expressing sounds that feel similar to the client's depressed or angry energy. Once the client feels a sympathetic vibration, he is more likely to resonate with the sound healer and to fall into alignment when she makes soothing and relaxing sounds.

The vibratory tools of sound, crystals, and essential oils are so powerful and so coherent that they can entrain the vibrations of depressed organs or tissues in the body. When just the right sound, crystal, or oil is chosen, it can remind the body of its own healthy harmonic resonance.

The same effect can be achieved when you strike a tuning fork that vibrates at 100 cps and bring it near another tuning fork of the same frequency, the second instrument will start vibrating without being struck. Then the two objects are in resonance with each other. External rhythms can also be used to affect the rate of the heart, respiration, and brain wave activity.

Every organ, bone, and cell has its own healthy resonant frequency. Sound healer Shari Edwards has the remarkable ability to hear these frequencies, and she has assigned a hertz frequency to each of the muscles, organs, and tissues of the body. Shari can also produce these sounds with her voice and has devised a machine that reproduces these sounds.

She and I were both teaching at a healing convention many years ago. When we met again, I had sustained an injury in which a boulder fell on my left thigh. It never fully healed, and my thigh had a large depression. I had the feeling that Shari could help so I explained my situation to her, and we went to her room to give it a try.

When I showed her my thigh, she reached out and placed her fingertips on the depression. Then she opened her mouth and a distinct sound came out. She used her machine to measure the frequency of the sound and it calibrated at a particular hertz. Then she looked it up in her booklet and sure enough, the sound she made was the exact frequencey for the thigh muscle.

Shari set me up with a pair of headphones and dialed in the sound I needed, and I sat there listening to the repetitions of this one sound. Half an hour later, she asked me to take off the headphones and stand up. We looked at my thigh, and we were both amazed and delighted to see that the depression was 80 percent gone.

Shari was applying the principle of *resonance* by invoking the sound of a healthy thigh muscle. When the less healthy muscle heard that sound, it presumably was stimulated to emulate its own healthy manifestation. When we hear a statement and respond by saying, "That resonates for me," we mean that it rings true, and it has a healthy harmonious vibration.

Shari was also using the principle of *entrainment* by encouraging my weak thigh muscle to lock in to the stronger healthy vibration of her machine. If you have a relatively weak voice, you have probably experienced entrainment while singing with stronger vocalists. It takes too much energy to sustain a tune at a weaker vibration, so your voice just naturally wants to lock in and sing along with the stronger voices.

**Bodily Harmony.** Dr. Peter Guy Manners works with sound in his medical practice in Worcester, England. He writes, "Experimentation indicates that human beings, as all objects, are radiating sound waves; therefore their fields are sonic fields."[49]

We are inclined to believe that reality is limited by what we experience with our five senses. It is difficult to believe that there are sounds we cannot hear and vibrations we cannot feel. Yet we know that infrared and ultraviolet light rays are invisible to our eyes, and there are subsonic and supersonic sounds that we cannot hear, and ultra high frequency (UHF) and extremely low frequency (ELF) vibrations we cannot feel.

The seawater crocodile senses electrical vibrations more than one hundred yards away. The shark has electrosensors covering its snout that sense the vibrations of creatures hiding under the sand. Sharks have a hearing-feeling sense (scientists call it a lateral line) through which they can sense the vibrations of moving prey.[50]

We are all vibrations, and every part of the body has a frequency. Dr. Manners defines harmony within the body and describes how to use sound to detect the source of bodily disharmony. He explains that just as each of us has our own unique shape and size, we each have our own distinct pattern, or collection of tones. "Within the human body any deviation from this harmony would result in ill health. . . . We can easily see that each organ will have its own sonic (or sound) field. If properly detected this should provide information on processes going on in a particular organ."[51]

Discoveries by Dr. Raymond Royal Rife in the 1930s show how potent the right tones can be for eliminating disease. He found that every cell has its own vibratory frequency, and every cell within a specific organ system has a common vibratory resonance. Rife is best known for his amazing microscope that magnifies living cells at hundred thousand magnifications. While observing the internal workings of a living human cell, he took a Ray-O-Vac tube and a frequency generator, and charged the cells with different frequencies. Eventually he found a resonance that exploded the cells.

Armed with this knowledge, Rife started curing cancer. For cancer of the breast, for example, he could take a biopsy of cancerous tissue and put it under the microscope and then observe the cells while he adjusted his frequency generator until the cells exploded. Once he knew the frequency that would obliterate the malignant cells, he put his patient next to the tube and directed it to her breast, and when the treatment was complete the cancer cells would be gone without affecting the rest of the breast or body.[52]

Perhaps Rife's work inspired the development of the German lithotripter, which translates as "stone crusher." This remarkable medical machine destroys kidney stones and gallstones by selectively attacking them with the appropriate sound resonance that mimics the sound frequency of the stones, causing them to break up. The machine passes high voltage electrical shock waves through a spark gap under water. The shock waves produce a compressive force, and the brittle stones start to crumble into small sand like particles that are passed out in the urine. Kidney, ureter, or bladder stones can all be treated in this painless procedure that takes two to three hours.[53]

Dr. William Tiller, a Guggenheim Fellowship recipient from Stanford University, writes in *Radionics, Radiesthesia and Physics*, that each gland of the body has its own healthy waveform, so one can scan the waveform of a gland to detect abnormalities. Then "if energy having the normal or healthy waveform of the gland is pumped into...the gland [it] will be driven in the normal or healthy mode." [54]

This helps explain why exercises in this section such as Toning for the Pain in Your Body and Toning with Bodywork (pages 164 and 165) are effective. Toning brings healthy waveforms into imbalanced or diseased tissues and organs, reawakening healthy vibrations within the body.

A physically sensitive healer can send out sounds, as a bat uses radar, to scan the wave field of each gland, checking for imbalances. Intuitively, he can find sounds to charge the glands with healthy energy, thereby restoring their healthy harmonic frequency.

Dolphins use sound for echolocation, and presumably this same skill enables them to detect abnormal areas of the body and to direct sound to those areas. This probably accounts for the seemingly miraculous healings that some people experience after swimming with dolphins. During my workshops on the Big Island of Hawaii, we swim and kayak with wild dolphins. No experience can compare with having these huge mammals voluntarily swim next to you in the ocean and look you in the eyes. The depth of their consciousness and compassion is undeniable.

Once I swam with a student who was pregnant though her belly was not noticeably enlarged. We were approached by nearly a dozen dolphins including two baby dolphins, swimming alongside their mothers. I was amazed to see a baby dolphin break away from its mother and swim in circles directly under this pregnant woman for at least five minutes. How did the baby dolphin—and its mother, who allowed it to swim alone—know that this woman was pregnant? Probably by sound, just as doctors use ultrasound to examine the fetuses of pregnant women.

**Whales and the Deep Sound Channel.** In 1943, two researchers at Columbia University exploded one pound of TNT in the Bahamas, and their receivers were able to detect the sound on the coast of West Africa, two thousand miles away. They were making use of the Deep Sound Channel used by whales and the U.S. Navy.

Sound passes almost five times faster in water than in air. There are four major horizontal thermal layers in deep seawater : 1) The *surface layer* undergoes daily changes in heating, cooling, and wind action. 2) The *seasonal thermocline* is affected by seasonal temperature changes. Temperature drops steadily with depth, and as the temperature falls, the speed of sound decreases (true also when sound travels through air). 3) The *permanent thermocline*, about a half mile below the surface, is only slightly affected by seasonal changes. 4) The *deep isothermal* layer has a nearly constant temperature. The increased water pressure causes sound to speed up (sound travels even faster, at 11,200 miles per hour, through solids than through water).

Where the bottom of the permanent thermocline (layer three) meets the top of the deep isothermic (layer four), sound travels thousands of miles horizontally with minimum signal loss. A sound wave traveling obliquely through this channel bends downward as the speed of sound decreases and bends upward when more water pressure causes the sound speed to increase.

During the 1950s, the U.S. Navy developed a Sound Surveillance System (SOSUS) that made use of this Sound Fixing and Ranging Channel (as they called it) to detect submarines. Christopher Clark, a biological acoustician at Cornell University, was permitted by the Navy to use the SOSUS receiver to listen to the voice patterns of blue, finback, minke, and humpback whales. Using a receiver in the West Indies, he could hear whales that were 1,100 miles away.[55]

Currently the U.S. Navy is trying to deploy sonar equipment known as LFAS (Low Frequency Active Sonar), an extended-range submarine-detection system over about 80 percent of the world's oceans. Each of the system's long array of transmitters generates 215 decibels (dB) of sound. After several hundred meters, the sound waves converge, boosting the noise level to an equivalent of more than 240 dB. Using this technology allows the navy to illuminate hundreds of thousands of square miles underwater at one time. This means that a low-frequency signal in the southern Indian Ocean, for example, can be detected off the West Coast of the United States.

In 1995, National Resources Defense Council demanded that the LFAS tests that had been conducted in complete secrecy be brought into compliance with environmental protection laws. The Pentagon agreed to conduct a full-scale study of environmental impacts. While many important questions were not addressed by the study, a thirty-two-year-old navy diver was briefly exposed to LFA sonar at a level of 160 dB (much less intense than the intended levels), and after twelve minutes he experienced severe symptoms, including dizziness and drowsiness. He was hospitalized and later relapsed, suffering memory dysfunction and seizures. Two years later he was being treated with antidepressant and anti-seizure medications.

The faintest audible sound has a sound pressure value of 0 dB. The loudest sound that the human ear can tolerate is about 120 dB. Normal conversation is 50 to 60 dB, heavy rock music goes up to about 110 dB, and pain threshold is about 125 dB.

In March 2000 in the Bahamas four different species of whales and dolphins were stranded on the beach just after the navy used extremely loud active sonar. Seven whales died, and analysis of their inner ears established with certainty that all but one of the whales suffered inner ear hemorrhaging.[56]

Many people are deeply concerned that the sounds being blasted throughout the oceans are damaging the delicate acoustic structures of the whales, as well as disrupting their mating and navigational channels.

## Toning

A tone is a distinct sound that maintains a constant pitch and is identifiable by its regularity of vibration. Toning is the sustained, vibratory sounding of single tones, often vowel sounds, without the use of melody, rhythm, or words. These sounds may cause vibrations that create overtones that reverberate in a way that can be highly penetrating.

Overtones are sounds that emanate from a single musical note and have a high frequency. Many overtones are higher than your ears' ability to hear, so these are called subliminal sounds and may explain why toning has the mysterious ability to put people into a trancelike state or to invoke profound emotions. This book will not teach you how to make overtones deliberately, but overtones tend to occur when you tone, especially in a group.

A tone may be high-pitched (having many vibrations per unit of time) and piercing or it may be low-pitched (having fewer vibrations) and soothing—or anything in between. A specific tone will have a fairly predictable effect on the person listening (and the person making the tone). High, piercing tones tend to speed up the heart, and low, soothing tones tend to slow it down. Harsh tones tend to create feelings of anxiety, while rich, mellow tones tend to elicit a sense of deep inner peace. Some tones stir up strong feelings, and others pull you out of your emotions, into a meditative state.

Pleasant low-pitched tones tend to produce a grounded, earthy sense of well-being. Low tones can help you get into your body and accomplish things. Pleasing, high-pitched tones can help release stress and day-to-day worries, producing a euphoric, deeply relaxed feeling.

Most people have heard the toning of the syllable OM, which is believed to create an energy of harmony and unity. Regardless of their religion, people tend to experience a quiet centeredness when OM is toned repeatedly, especially when it is done in a rich and sonorous voice.

During true spiritual expression, whether in a church or a synagogue, under a tree or on a mountain, people experience direct communion with their God or Creator. Toning, chanting, and droning are practices that virtually all cultures have used, particularly in their religious services. Whether you grew up chanting AMEN, OM, or AMEIN in your church, mosque, or synagogue, or whether your army, tribe, or football team made hollers or whoops, you have in all these ways experienced some form of toning.

We are seeing a spontaneous emergence of the intuitive use of sound. People are using toning for spiritual expression, enhancement of community feeling, and physical and emotional healing. People are listening to and expressing their inner voice in new and exciting ways: toning with tai chi, yoga, spontaneous dancing, lovemaking, toning at men's groups, and wailing at women's groups.

Even the cry of an infant can be a form of toning. Although infants are nonverbal, they can fully express distress, happiness, love, and anger. Simply through the use of vibratory sound, they persuade us to pick them up, feed them, comfort them, or change their diapers. If you have ever been an infant then you already know how to tone.

But most children in our culture learn how to censor their emotions, words, and every sound that comes out of their mouths. They learn to make only sounds that are socially acceptable. As a child, I was taught not to make loud noises of any kind: boisterous laughter, painful crying, and screaming with pleasure.

I grew up feeling secretive and shy about using my voice in a forceful and passionate way. I harbored a desire to sing, yet singing was only for people who had great voices. When I auditioned for the school chorus, I barely got in. I took two or three singing lessons, but my teacher was not terribly impressed. My main vocal achievements for the next twenty years consisted of improvised lullabies to my babies and then singing songs like "I've Been Working on the Railroad" during long trips in the car with my boys.

I didn't get over my fear of singing until I started toning. It's not necessary to have a beautiful or powerful voice to tone, and it's not possible to make mistakes!

The first person I heard tone was my friend Laeh Maggie Garfield, who wrote *Sound Medicine*. It was a loud, intense sound that shocked me. But it also vibrated deeply within me. I never imagined that I would be able to make such sounds or that I would want to!

The next time I heard toning was when I taught at a women's retreat in California, where I attended a workshop with Dhyani Ywahoo, author of *Voices of Ancestors*. She held a huge crystal in each hand and made powerful unearthly sounds that awakened something within me. It would be years before I could give myself permission to make such sounds.

But eventually I did. Then I helped others do the same. I find that it is easier for people who are not trained as singers to let themselves make uninhibited sounds than for singers who are trained to believe there is a right and a wrong way to make sounds.

I still felt shy about *sounding* (another word for *toning* or making improvised sounds) in public, but I would tone with my students as we made sounds for the chakras. Sometimes the whole room would reverberate with overtones bouncing off the walls and ceiling—as if there were a chorus of angels on the rooftop.

Gradually I overcame my shyness. The feedback I received about my toning was so positive that it gave me confidence. The sounding took on a life of its own. It seemed to have its own intelligence, and I learned to trust it. During meditations or talks or healings I would be overwhelmed by the desire to make sounds. I just had to open my mouth and the sounds would come pouring out of me. Eventually I produced a CD called *Altered States of Planet Earth* (see Resources). It combines my spontaneous sounds that I call Shamanic Sounding with Alejo's didjeridoo, a long instrument made originally by the Australian Aborigines by hollowing out a small tree.

**Toning with Laughter**. Laughter is a form of toning. One Zen master told his students that if they would say "HO! HO!" vigorously for five minutes each day, they would never die. According to Laurel Elizabeth Keyes, author of *Toning, The Creative Power of the Voice*, the *H* and *K* sounds such as *HI, HAH, HOH, HU, KAH* and *KOO*. stimulate the glandular system. They are produced by tightening the abdominal muscles and forcing the breath against the roof of the mouth, thereby creating strong vibrations in the adrenal, thymus, pituitary, and pineal glands. We conceptualize laughter as a repetition of *h* sounds such as *ha-ha-ha* or *he-he-he*.[57]

Norman Cousins provides yet another way of using laughter for healing in *Anatomy of an Illness*. He had a rare life-threatening disease, ankylosing spondylitis, characterized by a gradual deterioration of collagen, the fibrous substance that holds the body together through the connective tissue in every part of the body and particularly the spine.

Cousins was familiar with research showing that repeated stress leads to illness and disease. He reasoned that if distress causes disease, joy and laughter should cause healing, so he arranged to have funny movies and hilarious old TV programs shown throughout the day in his hospital room. He discovered that ten minutes of good belly-laughing provided a full two hours of pain relief. Eventually Cousins cured his disease with a combination of laughter and massive doses of vitamin C.[58]

**Abdominal Breathing**. Toning expands the abdomen and lower lungs, pushing stale air out of the lungs, enabling you to absorb more fresh oxygenated air. You don't need to have strong breath control, but since toning requires deep breathing, it contributes to health and a sense of peacefulness, helps eliminate the effects of stress, and can help prevent (and sometimes heal) heart disease, asthma, bronchitis, and senility.

Shallow breathing contributes to a lack of oxygen. The habit of shallow breathing begins in early childhood, when children are forced to be quiet, to be still, to hold back their feelings. When you're scared, you literally hold your breath. You don't let a single sound escape, not even a sigh. When you're afraid, angry, excited, or sad, you tend to take very shallow breaths, because taking a deep breath would expand your heart or abdomen, and that's where you hide those intense emotions. That's why children so often complain of tummy aches when they're emotionally upset, and why adults consume so many little tablets for indigestion.

American women rarely breathe from their abdomens, because they believe they look better with flat, rigid stomachs instead of relaxed, rounded ones. Women (and men) with rigid stomachs often have trouble with indigestion and may have trouble getting in touch with their feelings.

If you feel inhibited about making sounds, you're not alone. One way to overcome this resistance is to start humming. Follow the exercises and hum instead of toning. When you get comfortable with humming, make a louder hum. As you notice that nothing terrible happens, you'll be able to make increasingly louder sounds.

Here's an exercise to strengthen your diaphragm and give you better control of your breathing. Stand up, with your feet shoulder length apart. As you take a deep breath, feel your lower abdomen (below your navel) and then your upper abdomen (above your navel) expand, like a balloon. Your shoulders will rise slightly. Hold your breath to the count of five and then—without exhaling—contract your entire abdomen. Push it out again. Then exhale and relax your entire abdomen. Practice until you can do this easily Next, inhale as before and hold your breath. Contract your abdomen and push it out as before, then repeat. Exhale and relax your stomach. Continue practicing until you can contract and push out your abdomen ten times while holding your breath.

**How to Tone**. The human voice is one of our finest tools for healing the body and spirit. Yet it weighs nothing, costs nothing, and you don't even have to carry it in your pocket.

When you're ready to tone, you can stand, or sit upright in a firm chair with your feet on the ground, or sit on a cushion on the floor in the tailor or cross-legged position. Be sure your spine is straight. Relax your jaw (you might open and close your mouth a couple times, as if you were yawning). Inhale through your nose. Feel your lower and then upper abdomen expanding. Before they are fully expanded, feel your breath continue up into your lower and then upper lungs as they, too, expand. Your shoulders will rise slightly. Feel your shoulders relaxing.

Relax your jaw; just let it hang open. Release your breath through your mouth while making a long sustained sound, preferably a vowel sound. This is the tone. Allow the sound to continue as long as you exhale. When you run out of breath the sound will stop. Inhale deeply through your nose as you bring your breath all the way down to your lower abdomen. Continue this process for as long as you like.

It is not necessary to concentrate too much on taking complete breaths. After the first few breaths, just relax and enjoy the process. Here are some exercises you can experiment with:

- Tone a long vowel (A, E, I, O, or U) at a comfortably low pitch for as long as your breath allows. Repeat several times. Tone the same vowel at a medium pitch. Repeat several times. Tone the same vowel at a comfortably high pitch. Repeat several times. Do the same with a different vowel.

- Tone a syllable (a single uninterrupted sound formed by a vowel and one or more consonants such as "OM") at a comfortably low pitch for as long as your breath allows. Repeat several times. Tone the same syllable at a medium pitch. Repeat several times. Tone the same vowel at a comfortably high pitch. Repeat several times. Do the same with another syllable, such as "RA."

- Let go entirely and play like a kid. Beat on a tabletop, hit a cup with a spoon, or bang pots and pans together. Get silly. Loosen up.

- Make up a song in a pretend language that sounds Indian, Chinese, or Greek.

- Get a drum that gives off lots of reverberations. Hit the drum repeatedly and try to imitate or blend your tones with the sounds.

- Get a Tibetan bowl or a quartz crystal bowl or a tuning fork, and make spontaneous sounds or chant the following Tibetan or Egyptian sounds.

The Tibetans have a sound for each chakra that can be chanted individually, or you can chant all of them on one breath: *LAM* (first chakra), *VAM* (second), *RAM* (third), *YAM* (fourth), *HAM* (fifth), *OM* (sixth and seventh).

Dr. Mitch Gaynor, oncologist, has had excellent results reducing stress and pain for his patients by having them play a Tibetan or crystal bowl while chanting the Tibetan seed sounds.[59]

The ancient Egyptians had sounds that were later adopted by the Rosicrucians. In one exercise, *AUM* is repeated twice at a low pitch. Then *RAH* and *MA* are sounded at a high pitch. Then *AUM* is repeated twice at the same low pitch.[60]

When using toning during a healing session, your client will probably be lying down. If she wishes to participate in the toning, it's perfectly all right to tone while lying down, but she may prefer to stand or sit while toning, and then lie down again.

Most of this book is directed toward self-healing, but all the exercises can be used in a client-practitioner or friend-friend context. In this section I address the Sound Healer. With some of the exercises, such as Toning for the Pain in Your Body, your client may feel too inhibited to make his own sounds. Once you become proficient at making sounds for yourself, you may be able to tune in on your client's emotions and give voice to his feelings—which may inspire him to begin making sounds for himself. Most people feel less self-conscious after hearing someone else make outrageous sounds, because there is less fear of being judged.

If you sense that a client is holding onto an emotional sound that she cannot get in touch with, you might say, "I feel the impulse to make a sound, and it may not be very pleasant. Is that all right?" If she says "yes," then you can add, "Feel free to join me."

When sounds are released, memories often come flooding up into awareness, so be prepared to do counseling in conjunction with this work.

There are three basic sounds:

1) **Cleansing and Releasing**. These sounds express emotions and help release stress and tension. Moaning and groaning are cleansing sounds that come naturally when aches and pains and strong emotions are being released.

   High-pitched, penetrating sounds or even fierce screaming can help break up energy blockages that may have led to emotional and physical armoring. Sharp, intense sounds combined with sweeping gestures can purge negative energy. If you feel the impulse to make sounds for your client, go ahead and release those sounds. You may feel a blood-curdling, terrifying scream, and your client may be amazed to find herself joining you. This could go on for several minutes and might actually end in laughter! Releasing a scream that has been held in for decades can be a joyous, liberating experience.

Sounds can also be used to cleanse the energy in a room. When people are angry, brooding, and unable to release heavy emotions, they tend to leave negative energy behind. A dark cloud seems to hover in the energy field of the room, even after they are gone. The same technique can be used to clean the energy in a room.

Many people are reluctant to make "negative" sounds in a room, partly because they are afraid of leaving their "bad energy" behind. I have found that the opposite is true. Unexpressed emotions linger in the energy field of a person or a room, whereas even the "worst" emotions, when fully expressed (without causing harm to others), leave the energy revitalized.

While you are making releasing sounds for your client, you may see him twitch, jerk, or tremble briefly as negative thought patterns and holding patterns are released. Don't be alarmed; this is perfectly natural.

2) **Soothing and Relaxing**. These sounds bring body and spirit back into their natural harmony and alignment. Through toning, you can provide a soothing environment for the release of tension. Humming can be calming to the nervous system and may help your client take deeper breaths.

You may feel inspired to sing words of support and encouragement, or even to break into familiar bars of music or pop tunes. Trust the impulse; it often turns out to be surprisingly appropriate.

3) **Regenerative**. Sit in silence with your client and allow your energy to align with his, so that you can *feel* the resonance that he is lacking. This may happen spontaneously while you are talking or while he is toning. Once you feel the needed resonance, allow your voice to provide that sound. When regenerative sounds are for survival or for resolving sexual issues, they tend to be low and full-bodied (corresponding to sounds for the lower chakras). When they are for healing the emotional body, they usually fall in the mid-range (corresponding to the middle emotional chakras). When they are for opening to

spirituality, they tend to be high and ethereal (corresponding to the higher chakras).

You may notice tears rolling down your client's face. He may experience a wave of heat rushing over him, or a cool breeze. He may feel goose bumps on his skin. His heartbeat may slow down or increase. He may have a sensation of a great weight being lifted from his shoulders.

Sometimes—particularly toward the end of a session—you may have an impulse to sing silly songs: popular songs, hillbilly songs, rock and roll, sentimental songs. These often turn out to be just the right thing, and the laughter that follows may be just the right ending for your session.

## Emotional Release through Toning

The following exercises are specially designed to help you get in touch with your emotions. Toning is one of the most powerful tools for releasing pent-up, repressed emotions. Sound bypasses the intellect and has the inherent ability to trigger physical or emotional reactions: Your eyes and nose may water, phlegm may come up from your chest, you may cough, your sinuses may feel aggravated, you may feel tightness in your neck, shoulders, and chest, your heart may beat rapidly or feel painful, your body may twitch, you may feel dizzy or nauseous. Buried memories may come flooding into your consciousness.

These symptoms are signs that the toning is working for you, stirring up emotional and physical blockages that have been preventing you from breathing and living freely. If you are accustomed to holding in your feelings, you may be afraid that something terrible is going to happen if you lose control. Releasing control for a while can lead to becoming relaxed and healthy. Having too much control leads to illness, including heart attacks, high blood pressure, and arthritis.

Some people are afraid that once they open up, they'll become violent or crazy. I can assure you that I have never met anyone who became mentally or physically ill as a result of expressing their emotions. However, I have met innumerable people who became both mentally and physically ill as a result of *suppressing* their emotions.

Still, there is a fear—no matter how irrational—that once you open the box of repressed emotions and let them out, you will never get it closed again. After over thirty years of helping people with emotional release, the only problem I've seen occurs when people get scared and try to close the box.

If you are unaccustomed to releasing emotions, and if it is intensely disturbing to you, you may want to have someone present that you feel comfortable with, who can hold and comfort you if the need arises. *If you know that you have a lot of pain to release, and you're not sure that you can handle it—alone or with a friend—seek the help of a trained counselor or therapist, and ask this person to work with you as you do these exercises.*

There are other precautions you can take. Before you begin working, sit quietly and take ten deep breaths. Tell yourself, "I give myself permission to temporarily lose control. I will not do harm to myself or to anyone or anything else." Repeat this three times. It is like making a pact with your subconscious. I have never seen anyone violate such an agreement.

If you feel upset during or after these exercises, just sit quietly and bring ten deep breaths all the way down to your lower abdomen. Watch it expand each time you inhale. This will help to calm and ground you. People usually feel considerably lighter and better after doing these exercises. They breathe better, their sinuses open, and they feel empowered. Most people delight in discovering that they enjoy making sounds as their voices become stronger, fuller, and more vibrant.

If you would like to do these exercises but find that you just can't do them—if you can't even begin to open your mouth and make loud sounds—you may have been punished for being noisy when you were a child. Punishment can take the form of a harsh look or a strap. Very sensitive children respond to a sharp glance as if they'd been hit.

Even if you weren't punished, you may have internalized the idea that it is bad, naughty, inconsiderate, or obnoxious to make loud noises. For a child, it is a matter of survival to be accepted by her caregivers, so most children learn to behave in a way that is acceptable to adults. Even after we are grown, when we behave in ways that our caregivers did not approve of, it triggers that old fear of abandonment. So when someone asks you to make loud noises, even if you think it's a good idea, you may find that you simply can't do it.

One way to overcome this resistance is to start humming. Follow the exercises and hum instead of toning or groaning or making loud noises. When you get comfortable with humming, make a louder hum. As you notice that nothing terrible happens, you will be able to let yourself make louder noises.

The important thing is to *release* any pent-up feelings that you may have, and to *express* your emotions. As you're doing this, you may find yourself yawning, screaming, crying. Your body may jerk, shiver, or tremble. You may want to pound on the bed with your fists or stomp your feet. If you are standing, you may want to fall down on the mat. Just make sure you have plenty of padding under you.

Just let it happen. If your body is twitching and jerking, this is good. It means that your body is finally breaking free of its armoring, and you will probably feel much better afterward. Give yourself as much acceptance as you possibly can, and let yourself release whatever needs releasing. Exaggerate your sounds. If you notice that your voice is beginning to sound like a siren, make a loud siren noise. If you're starting to sound like a howling dog, then *become* a howling dog. If you sound like a baby crying, then become a baby calling out desperately for its mama. Don't worry about sounding silly. Try not to judge yourself.

Welcome the emotions, no matter how painful or how wonderful. Emotions that are pent-up are limiting or poisoning you. Instead of shying away from the exercise because it seems to be making things worse, try going more deeply into it; instead of doing it for five minutes, try it for ten. You may get worse before you get better, but this is almost certainly going to help. By the end of the session, you are likely to notice a distinct change for the better.

Dr. Elisabeth Kubler-Ross did groundbreaking work with teenagers in high schools where there were serious problems with violence. She persuaded certain school boards to put in soundproof screaming rooms with mattresses on the floors and walls, so kids could go in and beat the mats and scream their heads off. When students had a physical outlet for their emotional pain, they no longer needed to numb themselves with drugs and alcohol, and they had less need to be aggressive with other students. Screaming is a form of *sounding*—making uninhibited sounds without specific words.

Here is a story about how one young woman used sound to feel better.

Anna was an emotionally withdrawn and extremely overweight teenager. When she was feeling especially depressed, she found it comforting to turn on rock music. The worse she felt, the louder she turned up the music.

Rock stars are best loved when they are most outrageous. They wear crazy costumes, paint themselves wildly, do strange things to their hair, act out with blatantly childish behavior, and make loud, raucous music. They do everything that a teenager's parents tell them not to do.

We live in a spectator society, where most of us grow up watching television instead of getting out and living our lives. We watch others play sports instead of playing sports ourselves. We ask others to pray for us instead of praying for ourselves. Most of us expect others to think for us instead of thinking for ourselves. There are ways in which we get others to express our feelings instead of expressing them ourselves.

I taught Anna how to tone, and she was finally able to express the pain she felt at being emotionally abandoned by her mother. Once she gave herself permission to scream and yell, she no longer needed the rock stars to do it for her. As she released the pain, the sound went from meek to strong and full, and she was amazed by the power of her own voice.

Over the next few sessions, her voice grew stronger, and she noticed herself becoming more assertive, demonstrative, and out-going. She lost the compulsive need to keep feeding her face and stuffing down her emotions, and she dropped forty pounds in two months. Though she still enjoyed certain rock stars, she had no more interest in listening to intensely loud music.[61]

Adults, too, can benefit from some form of emotional release. When we are in stressful situations, we automatically start pumping adrenaline and other hormones for fight or flight. That adaptation served us in primitive times when we had to kill an enemy or run from attack. But in modern times, we become civilized and learn to suppress these instincts.

When you stifle your natural impulses, these hormones turn into toxins that get stored in your body and gradually build up to create chronic physical problems. I have no medical evidence of this, but I have helped innumerable people to relive traumatic incidents from childhood. When they can scream and curse and hit the mat, the incidents come back with perfect clarity, as if they happened yesterday.

The release of old repressed emotions enables clients to experience a sense of anticipation and joy in life they hadn't felt since they were infants. When they express and then let go of emotional pain that plagued them for years, their physical pain falls away. They stop drinking alcohol and using harmful medications, whether they are street drugs or pharmaceuticals.

Toning is a remarkable way of letting go of emotions that have become trapped in specific parts of the body. It is also a way of restoring harmony so that the ailing part can find its natural interrelationship with the whole body, allowing the energy to flow freely.

As the preverbal infant so eloquently demonstrates, sounds can express every nuance of human emotion. If young children are not repressed, you can see in them a perfect demonstration of the art of emotional release through sounding. When a child is sad, she will cry, wail, or moan. When a child is happy, she will sing, shout, and giggle.

These sounds may be distressing to adults who seek to create a harmonious atmosphere. Since we are constantly bombarded by sounds we cannot control, it's natural to want to eliminate the ones that we *can* control. Since we're bigger than our children, it's tempting to tell them to be quiet. But it is damaging to suppress a child's natural emotional expression. This doesn't mean that children should be encouraged to yell and scream and be inconsiderate of others. But there are times when emotional outbursts are appropriate, and a discerning adult will be able to recognize such times.

A wide variety of new therapies have emerged to help adults relive incidents from their childhood when they were not allowed to express their emotions. Sounding is one of these techniques. Allowing children (and adults) to release emotions through sound and movement can contribute to their emotional, mental, and physical health, as the following story from my book, *The Healing Voice*, clearly illustrates.

Alana and her twelve-year-old daughter, Lizzy, were driving home on a Friday night. Coming around the bend on the freeway, they saw a car about a half block ahead of them, making a dangerous U-turn in the middle of the road. The car was unable to complete the turn and Alana crashed into it.

Checking to see that neither she nor Lizzy was hurt, Alana got out of her car, still shaking from the shock and the impact, and went to the man to see if he was all right. Fortunately, there were no casualties, but both cars were demolished.

Alana felt proud of her composure as she waited for the police to arrive, trying to comfort poor Lizzy, who was sobbing uncontrollably. When the police drove up and started questioning Alana, Lizzy ran into the field alongside the car, screaming and hollering. It was extremely annoying to Alana, but she was committed to allowing her daughter to express her feelings—as long as she wasn't doing anything to harm anyone.

They got a ride home, and one hour after the accident, Lizzy returned to normal. Alana, on the other hand, discovered that she had severe whiplash in her left shoulder. This pain continued for months, until she came to me. I used light hypnosis to help her relive the accident, and she finally touched the true source of her pain: the utter fear of losing her child, and her life. I encouraged her to express this fear in sound, and she belted out a scream of sheer terror.

Through screaming, Alana was finally able to express and release her emotional pain, and the old program of having to brace herself for the impact. Her body had become frozen in a posture of tension since the powerful message she had sent to her muscles and tissues to be in a state of ready alertness. The scream was a message to her subconscious mind that the impact had, in fact, occurred, and now it was time to release.

The whiplash pain diminished over the next two weeks. If Alana had not been so civilized, she might have followed her daughter's example and released the pain immediately—or when she came home from the accident—and saved herself months of suffering.[62]

## Toning Exercises

Groaning and Moaning. This is a short emotional release exercise that you can do while you're in the shower or driving on a back-country road. A shower is ideal, because the water (preferably cool or cold water) is continuously bathing your electromagnetic aura and literally showering you with healthy negative ions. This is an excellent way to start the day or to wind down after work or after an argument or any stressful encounter. It gives you an opportunity to express your feelings without doing harm to anyone.

Start out by thinking about all the nasty things that have happened to you in the last week or month. Really get into it. Scrunch up your mouth and eyes and make ugly, disgusting faces like a six-year-old. Give yourself permission to be gross. Begin making low, groaning, moaning sounds. Feel sorry for yourself. Exaggerate it. Dramatize your feelings. Make loud, complaining, disgusting noises. Let your voice dredge up all the frustration, annoyance, and grief that you feel about anyone or anything.

After doing this for a while, your voice will go into a higher register. It may go up and down. As you release tension and begin to feel better, your voice will tend to go higher for longer. At some point, you will feel a definite release and a leveling off. You may sigh or tone a long note. You will know when you are finished. This typically takes five to ten minutes, but varies from person to person (the first or second time may take much longer). Just continue until you feel complete.

**Toning for the Pain in Your Body.** Focus on a painful part of your body and think of three words that describe the pain. Write them down. Think of a metaphor for the pain such as, "My hip feels like a rusty machine with the gears locked." Write that down.

Now give a sound to the first feeling. If the sound doesn't come spontaneously, begin by toning on a low note and slowly raise the pitch until you find a tone that resonates with the pain. Continue making sounds until you feel a release, as if you've given yourself an inner massage. This may take five to ten minutes or more with each feeling.

Here is how the exercise worked with one of my clients. John had a pain in his shoulders. His three words were: "Tight . . . scrunched . . . heavy." I wrote these down and then I asked him for a metaphor by saying, "It feels like. . . ?" He responded, "It feels like I'm carrying the whole world on my shoulders." I wrote this down. Then I read the first word aloud. I asked him to move around and make sounds to express feeling tight. He had a little trouble doing that, so I told him to, "Begin by making low sounds and slowly raise the pitch until you find a sound that feels tight. It might be a weird sound." Then I realized that he might feel self-conscious making such a sound, so I offered to demonstrate. I went into my own body, and it wasn't too hard to remember having a tightness in my own shoulders. I scrunched up my shoulders and made a strange gutteral sound that seemed to express the tightness. We both laughed and then it was easier for him. He rolled his head around on his neck and opened his mouth and made a powerful *OOOO* sound, which he continued to make until he felt a release.

He did a similar process with word "scrunched," this time making little barking sounds. With the word "heavy" he leaned over in a stooped position like an old man and made deep gutteral groans of pain. When this was complete, he stood up much straighter than before.

I asked him to make sounds for "I'm carrying the whole world on my shoulders." Suddenly his chin jutted forward and his shoulders came up again as he made short, fast panting sounds. He did this for several minutes, then shook himself off like a dog coming out of the water. "My God!" he exclaimed. "I feel totally different! The pain is gone. I never get that much relief from a massage."

This exercise works so effectively because it gives our bodies and voices an opportunity to express the pain, resentment, and frustration that we normally suppress. It's a great relief to be absolutely authentic. It takes a load off your shoulders.

**Toning with Bodywork.** It is rewarding to give yourself permission to make sounds while you are giving or receiving a massage, or any kind of bodywork. This section is directed to the masseuse, but the person receiving the work will also benefit from making sounds.

As I said earlier, there are three basic sounds: 1) cleansing and releasing, 2) soothing and relaxing, and 3) regenerative. Sounds may be released through the mouth into the air while you are massaging your client, or—if you want to direct the sound to a particular part of the body—you can cup your hands to create a kind of megaphone, with the mouthpiece at the circle formed by your thumbs and index fingers. Place your clasped hands directly on the painful part of your client's body and put your mouth to the mouthpiece, toning directly into the body. Some practitioners prefer to tone with their lips about a half inch from the body or to tone through the clothing or through a piece of cloth placed on the body.

Ted came to me because he had a serious case of lethargy and depression. Ordinarily I would begin by encouraging him to talk about what had been happening in his life, particularly the events preceding the feelings of depression. On this occasion, he had barely started talking when I had an impulse to press on his stomach. Asking for and receiving his permission, I started kneading the area around his solar plexus. Following my intuition, I found myself making gagging sounds, pushing firmly on his abdomen and gagging repeatedly (cleansing and releasing).

Ted broke into intense heaving sighs and released a well of tears (his own cleansing and releasing). "I've been feeling nauseous lately," he explained. "I'm feeling sick to my stomach about my family situation." He explained that his grown son wanted to come and live with him.

Though there was plenty of room in his house, it felt like an invasion of his privacy. Once he got in touch with his gut feelings, he realized that he wanted his son to make other arrangements.

I asked Ted to lie down, and I placed my hand gently on his solar plexus, mentally directing blue light to the area as I toned *UU* several times (soothing and relaxing). Then I directed yellow light to the same area as I toned *AOM* (regenerative). (See Visualization and Color Breathing, page 108.)

When I saw Ted two weeks later, he said that his depression "evaporated" after our session. "I had a great talk with my son, and it felt good to acknowledge my own needs, and my son seemed to respect me for that. It seems to be changing the whole dynamic of our relationship."

Another example involves a sixty-five-year-old man who got a new weed-trimmer and spent all afternoon enthusiastically whacking weeds. By evening, the muscles in his right forearm were so traumatized that he could barely make a fist, and his energy was completely depleted. The next morning he didn't feel any better, so he came to see me.

I asked if I could massage his forearm. He agreed, and as I worked on loosening up the muscles I seemed to be mentally reaching into that part of his arm. Feeling a strong impulse to make a high-pitched sound, after receiving his permission, I gave voice to the sound that seemed to be stuck in there. Suddenly I realized that the sound I was making was probably on the same pitch as the weed trimmer (which he confirmed).

By giving voice to that sound, I was initiating a process of cleansing and releasing. Then I made a low, deep tone as a kind of antidote, to calm his energy (soothing and relaxing). Within a few minutes, the pain was gone and much of his strength restored. The next day he called to say that his arm was fine and he was feeling energetic again.

Sounding can be combined with bodywork in a variety of ways. Find a friend who is open-minded. Offer to give her a massage in exchange for being able to experiment with sound. Before the massage, ask permission to make absolutely any sounds you feel like making. Encourage your friend to do the same. When you finish the session, sit down and give each other feedback about how it felt to work together.

Most people enjoy this kind of massage, but if your friend does not respond favorably, don't be discouraged. It's a matter of personal preference. Just find another friend and try again.

**Group Toning.** I find the following passage from Barbara Marciniak's book, *Bringers of the Dawn*, to be accurate and inspiring:

> When groups of you make sound together, you create an ambience for yourselves. You allow certain energies to play the instrument of your bodies. You let go of preconceived ideas and allow different melodies and energies to use your physical bodies as opportunities to represent themselves on the planet. . . .
>
> Sound is going to evolve. Now human beings can become the instruments for sound through toning. . . . They allow energies to use their physical bodies to make a variety of sounds that they do not direct or attempt to control the range of. Spirit plays, and human beings simply observe the attendance of the symphony that they and all the others are performing. It is quite profound. . . .
>
> One of the things that is important for utilizing these harmonics is to be very silent once the harmonics are complete. The harmonics alter something; they open the door. Certain combinations of sounds played through the human body unlock information and frequencies of intelligence. Being silent for a long period after the harmonics allows human beings to use their bodies as devices to

receive and absorb the frequencies and to use the vehicle of breathing to take them into an ecstatic state.

When you tone with others, you have access to the group mind that you did not have prior to making the sound. It is a gigantic leap in consciousness. *The key word is harmony.* When the entire planet can create a harmonic of thought, the entire planet will change. . . .

Those who are rewarded with the understanding that they are called to use sound as part of their work and who recognize that call and respond to it will evolve at a rapid pace. Those of you evolving at this rate will be called one day to represent many people, to represent world gatherings of consciousness, and to change the available frequency with your sound.[63]

Whenever a group is gathered—for a party, meditation, workshop, or just a family gathering—you have the potential to enjoy group toning. It is not necessary that people have previous experience at toning, though it does make it easier.

Toning is a way of adding another dimension to whatever is already happening. When I gather with my friends, we will sometimes form a circle and tone together. Joining hands in a circle helps bring our energies together, with our right palms down (because most of us give out energy from our right hands) and our left palms up (because most of us tend to receive from our left sides). This creates a weaving of energy within the circle, in which each participant is both giving and receiving energy.

Choose one person to facilitate and then decide what kind of toning to do. There are three primary choices: 1) toning simultaneously, with everyone beginning each tone at the same time and holding it as long as possible and then waiting until everyone is ready to begin the next tone; 2) toning simultaneously, with everyone beginning each tone at the same time and holding it only until most of the other people have stopped; 3) starting whenever you feeling inspired, holding the tone as long as you wish, and then starting up again so the tones of different people overlap.

The first two methods tend to create overtones, which can be extremely rich and rewarding. The overtones give the sensation of other voices echoing or reverberating off of the original voices. The third method keeps the sound going without pause, which can create an intense and pleasing effect. In any case, eventually the group will find its own completion and the tones will taper off. Your group may sound for just a few or you may go on for ten minutes or more, creating uncanny improvised harmonies.

Here is one possible format.

**Expressing Your Essence.** Everyone stands in a circle with their hands at their sides. Then say to the group: "Picture white light above your head. Inhale and bring in that light through your nose, to your heart. Exhale through your mouth and release tension. Do this ten times." Pause.

Ask everyone to go within and notice the following: "How does your body feel? Are you fatigued? Is your body tight anywhere? Do you feel loose and joyful? In a minute, I'm going to ask you to make sounds to express your feelings. These might not be pleasant sounds. Just use your voice to release the tensions of the day. Feel free to groan or moan or sigh. Just let go and release for a few minutes." Ask everyone to turn around and face away from the center of the circle. Pause until they do this.

"All right. Go!" Pause for a few minutes to let people release. Be sure to do this yourself.

"Okay. Turn around and face the center of the circle. Let's be quiet now. Breathe deeply. Inhale and bring your breath all the way down to your lower abdomen. Feel your abdomen expanding like a balloon. Let your breath be so strong that your neighbor can hear it." Pause for a minute.

"Now join hands, with the right palm down and the left palm up." Pause to do this. "Go inside and feel your essence. You might experience it as energy or color. Now express your essence with sound. Don't think about it; just open your mouth and let the sound come out. As you do this, listen to the group sound, and see if you can bring your sound in harmony with the group sound."

Continue this for at least a few minutes, until the group finds its own harmony. If the energy is good, you may want to continue for a long time.

**Prayers for World Peace.** Using crystals with this meditation is not necessary, but if you have them, do not underestimate their power to amplify your thoughts and your tones and to help create the kind of reality that you are projecting. Place a projector crystal where it can be seen by the group. This is a single-terminated crystal that stands up by itself, without support. The projector gathers and holds energy and then directs that energy into the noosphere (the atmosphere of ideas that surrounds the planet). During the meditation, each person can hold their individual single-terminated crystal pointing toward the projector crystal, charging it with their thoughts and energies.

If there is ample time, begin with the exercise Toning for the Chakras (page 171) until you reach the crown chakra. If time is short, begin by toning *OM*, with each person finding the pitch that feels best. Then sit in silence for at least five minutes.

If you're praying for peace in a particular part of the world, visualize a map of that area (someone might bring a map and you can look at it before you begin). Send the green light of love with the sound *AH* for the heart chakra. Then send calming blue light and the tone *UU*.

Visualize those who are in power. Tone *AH* for the heart chakra and send the pink light of love, which melts away aggression.

For those who are suffering from death or loss, who are in crisis, or who are hungry, flood their hearts with pink and green light and send the tone *AH*. Send blue and tone *UU* to calm them and ease their pain.

You can also use the Seed Sounds described under the Cultural and Spiritual Uses of Sound on page 120. Experiment with using these sounds to increase and decrease energies.

Follow your heart and continue your meditation in whatever way feels appropriate. Before you close, encourage everyone to speak from his or her heart and express appreciation aloud. When we remember to give thanks, we attract miracles.

If you used Toning for the Chakras in the beginning, come back down through the chakras, with one tone for each chakra.

When your meditation is complete, make a circle, join hands, and let everyone hold their clasped hands up in the air and shake their hands all together and cry out, "Be happy!" or "Be real!" whatever feels good to you. It is an excellent way to end a meeting.

## Toning for the Chakras

You can derive great benefit from using your voice to vibrate and strengthen your own chakras. You can also tone for others, to energize their chakras. According to Dr. Alfred A. Tomatis, we charge the brain when we speak or sing, and the greatest charge comes from the higher frequencies. So the most effective way to charge the brain, which in turn charges the whole body, is by using a rising curve in your sound.[64] The exercise below follows that pattern.

When toning for a given chakra, place your fingertips lightly over that area. Begin by trying the tones that I give in the chart, then experiment with different notes and tones until you find a sound that causes a vibration beneath your fingertips.

There are many systems of toning. For the sake of musicians, I have given the C major scale as a guideline for moving through the chakras, beginning with middle C at the tailbone, and ending with B at the crown. If you are not a musician, don't be intimidated by this. The main guideline is that—as you go up through the chakras—each tone should be higher than the previous one (and not necessarily by just one note). In my practice, I do not necessarily use the scale of C major, and I use different notes at different times. But I always use low notes for the low chakras, and progressively higher notes for the higher chakras.

The most important factor in toning for the chakras is to make a tone (the combination of a sound and note) that—for you—vibrates the chakras. There are no right or wrong tones, and you do not have to be musically inclined to be good at toning. People who have no ear for music have wonderful results.

As you do this exercise, you will be combining toning with Color Breathing, as described in Part 2. The following chart gives the color, note and tone for each chakra, and an "as in" word to clarify how the tone should sound (example: E as in red).

| Chakra | Color | Note | Tone | As In |
|--------|-------|------|------|-------|
| First | red | C | E | red |
| Second | orange | D | OO | home |
| Third | yellow | E | AOM | amen/home/mom |
| Fourth | green/pink | F | AH | amen |
| Fifth | blue | G | UU | blue |
| Sixth | indigo | A | MM | mom |
| Seventh | violet | B | EE | glee |

# PART 5

# Healing with Aromatherapy

From Tom Robbins's *Jitterbug Perfume*:

Of our five senses, the one most directly connected to memory is the sense of smell. Although man has become increasingly visual in his orientations. . . sight simply cannot compete with smell when it comes to the ability to awaken memory. Memories associated with scent are invariably more immediate and more vivid than those associated solely with visual imagery or sound. . . .

Scent is the last sense to leave a dying person. After sight, hearing, and even touch are gone, the dying hold on to their sense of smell. . . .

Fragrance is a conduit for our earliest memories, on the one hand; on the other, it may accompany us as we enter the next life. In between, it creates mood, stimulates fantasy, shapes thought, and modifies behavior. It is our strongest link to the past, our closest fellow traveler to the future. Prehistory, history, and the afterworld, all are its domain. Fragrance may well be the signature of eternity.[1]

We all respond strongly to aromas. Perfumes are among the most expensive commodities on earth. Condensing aroma-producing flowers into highly concentrated substances yields both perfumes and essential oils. When oils are prepared with great care, they vibrate at a high frequency. Some oils even have antibiotic properties. Essential oils are so effective that in France there are hospitals that heal primarily with essential oils.

The definition of aromatherapy is a therapy using only the essential oils from plants, as distinct from herbalism, which uses all parts of the plant (and therefore includes aromatherapy), and from perfumery, which is non-therapeutic.[2]

## History of Aromatherapy

According to records dating back to 4500 B.C.E., the Egyptians used balsamic substances (fragrant resins exuded from certain trees) medicinally and in religious rituals. Imhotep, the Grand Vizier (a government official) for King Zeser of Egypt (2780–2720 B.C.E.), popularized the use of oils, herbs, and aromatic plants as medicinals. In 1817, an 870-foot-long Egyptian document was discovered and dated to 1500 B.C.E. The Ebers Papyrus gives specific formulations used by the alchemists and high priests of Egypt for blending aromatic substances. Some were crushed and steeped in olive oil.

In 1922, the tomb of King Tutankhamon (ruled circa 1358– 1340 B.C.E.) was discovered almost intact, and 350 liters of oil were found in alabaster jars. The containers were sealed with plant wax, and the liquefied oil was in excellent condition.[3] The Egyptians perfected the art of embalming, using aromatic resins and essential oils to prevent the rot and decay of flesh. The priests correctly predicted that the bodies would last at least three thousand years.[4]

The Buddhist king, Ashoka (third century B.C.E.), took great pride in his medicinal garden, which produced many remedies, including aromatics that became famous throughout Asia and are still used in Indian Ayurvedic medicine.[5]

The Bible is full of references to spices, oils, and strong-smelling herbs, as seen in the love songs of the Old Testament's poetic *Song of Solomon*:

1:2–3 Because of the savour of thy good ointments thy name is as ointment poured forth, therefore do the virgins love thee.

1:12–14 While the king *sitteth* at his table, my spikenard sendeth forth the smell thereof.

A bundle of myrrh *is* my well-beloved unto me; he shall lie all night betwixt my breasts.

My beloved *is* unto me *as* a cluster of camphire in the vineyards of Engedi.

3:6 Who *is* this that cometh out of the wilderness like pillars of smoke, perfumed with myrrh and frankincense, with all powders of the merchant?

4:6, 10, 12–14,16 Until the day break, and the shadows flee away, I will get me to the mountain of myrrh, and to the hill of frankincense.

How fair is thy love, my sister, my spouse! how much better is thy love than wine! and the smell of thine ointments than all spices!

Thy plants are an orchard of pomegranates, with pleasant fruits; camphire, with spikenard,

Spikenard and saffron; calamus and cinnamon, with all trees of frankincense; myrrh and aloes, with all the chief spices.

Awake, O north wind; and come, thou south; blow upon my garden, that the spices thereof may flow out. Let my beloved come into his garden, and eat his pleasant fruits.

Obviously all of these aromas were familiar, and their use in ointments as well as in aphrodisiacs was well known. The New Testament contains a familiar story in Matthew 2:1-2, 11:

Now when Jesus was born in Bethlehem of Judea in the days of Herod the king, behold, there came wise men from the East to Jerusalem,

Saying, Where is he that is born King of the Jews? for we have seen his star in the east, and are come to worship him. . .

And when they were come into the house, they saw the young child with Mary his mother, and fell down, and worshipped him: and when they had opened their treasures, they presented unto him gifts; gold, and frankincense, and myrrh.

This was an apt gift for the baby boy who was born in a stable and was about to go on a long journey through the desert to escape from Herod. Frankincense strengthens high immune-system properties, and myrrh prevents the growth of bacteria.

When the physicians of Greece traveled along the Nile, they brought home the healing knowledge of the Egyptians. The ancient Greeks discovered that the aromas of certain flowers had a stimulating and refreshing effect, while the aromas of others were more relaxing and soothing. Greek soldiers carried an ointment of myrrh into battle to treat their wounds. Knowledge of the oils was shared with the Romans and Celts.

After the fall of Rome around 476 C.E., some physicians fled to Constantinople, taking their books and herbal knowledge with them. In the Byzantine Empire, perfume became popular, as did the medical use of aromatic oils. Avicenna (980–1037 C.E.), a great Arab physician, described more than eight hundred plants and their effects on the body. He is often credited with inventing the still, but in 1975 a perfectly preserved distillation unit made of fired terra-cotta was discovered in a town in Pakistan, at the foot of the Himalayas, dating back to 4000 B.C.E. Nevertheless, Avicenna did improve the still in the eleventh century, and the "perfumes of Arabia" (essential oils) became famous in Europe.[6]

During the great plague of the thirteenth and fourteenth centuries, some of the spice traders from the East became grave robbers. They protected themselves from the sickness by rubbing their bodies with oils such as pine, frankincense, balsam, clove, cinnamon, rosemary, and garlic.[7] Combinations of these oils are now known as "thieves' oil" and are popular for immunity from disease while traveling. Many of those oils are now recognized as powerful disinfectants, insecticides, and insect repellents. Others are effective bactericides and antiviral agents.

In the sixteenth century, the perfume industry in Provence, France, began producing essences of lavender and aspic (a species of lavender). By the beginning of the seventeenth century, most of the useful essences of Europe and the Near East had been discovered.[8]

With the invention of the printing press in the sixteenth century, recipes for producing oils were published in popular books called herbals. Methods for preparing infused oils, aromatic waters, decoctions, and herbal infusions became common knowledge. Women made herbal sachets to protect their linen from moths, and people wore little bags of aromatic herbs and garlic to ward off infections and the plague.[9]

Herbs and "simples" again became popular among women throughout Europe, as midwives and "witches" were sought after for their healing abilities. Then, during the industrial revolution, people moved to the cities, abandoning their gardens and losing the knowledge of simple herbs. By 1896 chemical science gained momentum as the therapeutic properties of plants became isolated and synthesized.[10]

In 1920, aromatherapy rose like a phoenix from the ashes when a French chemist, René-Maurice Gattefossé, suffered a third-degree chemical burn on his hand and forearm while working in his family's perfume company. As the story goes, his colleague was just bringing in a container of lavender oil from the cooler, and thinking it was cold water, the chemist plunged his arm into the vat. To his amazement, the pain subsided. With subsequent applications of the oil, the burn healed without a trace of scarring. Gattefossé developed the use of essential oils in dermatology and coined the term *aromatherapie* in a scientific paper, publishing a book by the same name in 1928.[11]

Gattefossé shared his experience a friend in Paris, Dr. Jean Valnet. They experimented with the essential oils, and the results were impressive. During World War II, Valnet was called to serve as a doctor in the French Army at the China Wall. When he ran out of medications, he fell back on the oils. To his amazement, he was able to reduce and even stop infections, thus saving many lives.

Later Valnet successfully treated psychiatric patients with herbs and oils. He wrote about this in a book called *Aromatherapie*, which was translated into English as *The Practice of Aromatherapy*.[12] Valnet's work was developed further by Dr. Paul Belaiche and Dr. Jean Claude Lapraz. Their laboratory research showed that essential oils contain antiviral, antibacterial, anti-fungal, and antiseptic properties, and have the ability to increase oxygen in the body.[13]

In the late 1950s aromatherapy was being practiced medicinally in France, and essential oils were being prescribed and stocked by pharmacies. Then an Australian woman married a French homeo-path, Dr. Maury, and together they researched the oils and used them medicinally. Marguerite Maury opened aromatherapy clinics in Paris, England, and Switzerland.

She was allowed to teach beauty and massage therapy, but they could not treat medical conditions. Nor could they select their own oils because those blends were kept secret for commercial reasons. Eventually aromatherapy spread to Norway and Denmark and began to develop in the United States, Canada, Australia, New Zealand, South Africa, and Middle and Far Eastern countries.[14] Currently essential oils are used by doctors in France, who practice complementary medicine (see Glossary). Doctors in other countries, however, still regard the oils merely as health and beauty aids.

In the 1980s Gary Young, a California naturopath, became impassioned about using high-quality essential oils for therapeutic purposes. He studied in Switzerland, France, England, and Israel.[15] A brilliant entrepreneur, he developed his own line of oils, Young Living. In his zealous promotion of his oils, he spread the knowledge of aromatherapy throughout the United States.

## Spiritual & Magical Uses of Aromas

Burning incense is a time-honored tradition. Herbs have been burned in both the East and the West as part of most major religions. Egyptian priests formulated the aromas that Pharaohs used in times of prayer, war, and love. Statues of each of the gods had a particular fragrance with which they were anointed.

The word perfume comes from the Latin *per fumum*, which means "through the smoke." The wisdom of burning herbs that have bactericidal effects is obvious when groups of people gather, especially during plagues and epidemics. Frankincense (real incense) is still burned in Catholic churches. Many Native Americans burn sage and sweetgrass during ceremonies. Some hospitals in France diffuse thyme and rosemary as disinfectants.[16] In the 1960s at the University of California at Berkeley, branches of eucalyptus were strewn along the edges of the lecture rooms during outbreaks of fleas.

The Old Testament describes a special ointment that the Jews used for their sacred ark and tabernacle. "The Lord spake unto Moses" with specific instructions about the sacred use of incense and preparation of holy oil:

And thou shalt make an altar to burn incense upon: of [meadows] wood shalt thou make it.

And Aaron shall burn thereon sweet incense every morning...

And when Aaron lighteth the lamps at even, he shall burn incense upon it, a perpetual incense before the Lord throughout your generations.

Ye shall offer no strange incense thereon...

Moreover the Lord spake unto Moses, saying,

Take thou also unto thee principal spices, of pure myrrh five hundred *shekels,* and of sweet cinnamon half so much, even two hundred and fifty *shekels,* and of sweet calamus two hundred and fifty *shekels.*

And of cassia five hundred *shekels* after the shekel of the sanctuary, and of olive oil an hin:

And thou shalt make it an oil of holy ointment, an ointment compound after the art of the apothecary; it shall be an holy anointing oil.

And thou shalt anoint the tabernacle of the congregation therewith, and the ark of the testimony...

Upon man's flesh shall it not be poured, neither shall ye make *any other* like it, after the composition of it; it is holy, and it shall be holy unto you.

Whosoever compoundeth any like it, or whosoever putteth any of it upon a stranger, shall even be cut off from his people.

Exodus 30:1,7–9, 22–26, 32–33

Translated into a modern recipe, a shekel is about one-half ounce and a hin is about one and one-half gallons, so this would be like saying that a holy ointment (which should be used only by Jews and only for anointing their most sacred objects) would be prepared by combining the following.

16 pounds pure myrrh
8 pounds sweet cinnamon
8 pounds sweet calamus
16 pounds cassia
1½ gallons olive oil

## Science of Aromatherapy

Let's begin with a brief review of how the brain and nose work together. Then we can look at scientific and medical research in the field of aromatherapy, including Bruce Tainio's innovative work with the frequencies of essential oils.

### Olfactory Anatomy

Paul MacLean, former director of the Laboratory of the Brain and Behavior at the United States National Institute of Mental Health, developed a model of the human brain in which each of the three layers or brains are believed to have been established in response to evolutionary need. No one knows exactly how the brain works, but this is an appealing theory.

The **reptilian complex** was believed to have evolved first. It is made up of the brain stem and cerebellum. The brain stem coordinates the basic automatic survival functions of digestion, reproduction, circulation, and breathing. It also governs the fight-or-flight response to stress. The cerebellum controls movement.

According to MacLean's theory, the second brain that evolved is the **limbic system**, which includes the amygdala and hippocampus. It is about the size of a walnut, though the size of a woman's limbic system is larger than that of a man's. The amygdala is the center of emotions and it associates emotions with events. The hippocampus converts information into long-term memory and memory recall. The limbic system relates to food, sex, and smell. It controls appetite and sleep cycles. It motivates us to approach or avoid people or events. When this center is overactive it seems to lead to feelings of negativity, depression, and lack of motivation.

The third brain to evolve is the **cerebral cortex** or **neocortex**, which comprises five-sixths of the total brain. It is the center of language, speech, writing, and logic. It contains two specialized centers for voluntary movement and processing sensory information.

All three parts of the brain function simultaneously, but one part tends to predominate at any given time. The interconnections make things interesting. When the neocortex communicates with the limbic system, you have that challenging interface between thought, memory, and emotions, and motivation for voluntary action.

The olfactory system is the only one of the five sensory systems that goes directly from the sensory organ (the nose) to the part of the brain where the sensation is processed. The senses related to sight, hearing, touch, and taste must first pass through the thalamus at the base of the cerebrum before they are registered in different parts of the brain. This helps to account for the powerful emotional impact that smell has upon us.[17]

The olfactory lobe is located under the frontal lobe. In most vertebrates it is a distinct extension of the cerebral hemisphere, but in human beings it is long and slender, with anterior and posterior lobules. A mucous membrane covers the bony extension on each side of the nose, and there is an olfactory membrane on each of these mucous membranes. These olfactory membranes are so tiny that they can only be seen through an electron microscope on high magnification, yet they contain about 800 million nerve endings for processing and detecting odors.[18]

About twenty nerves make up the first cranial or olfactory nerves, and extend from under the surface of the olfactory bulb,[19] back toward the midbrain. These nerves pass between the pituitary and pineal glands, carrying impulses directly to the amygdala, which is the memory center that stores and releases emotional trauma. Only odor has a profound effect upon this gland,[20] which helps explain why certain aromas can "calm the savage beast."

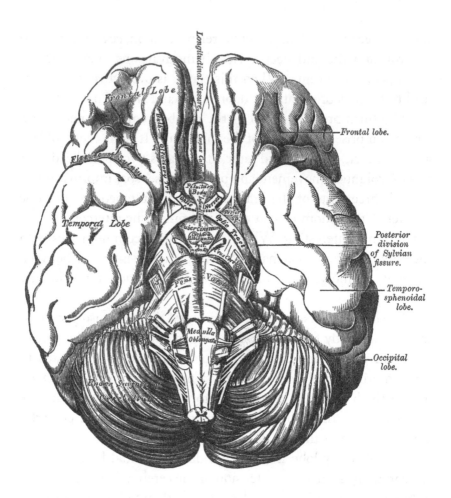

Essential oils penetrate the body through the skin, nasal passages, lungs, and gastrointestinal tract, and then they are carried through the blood and lymph.[21]

## Research in Aromatherapy

In European countries, essential oils are used in clinics and hospitals, and a wide selection of high quality oils are commonly sold in drugstores. Dr. Valnet writes about how "phyto- and aroma-therapy have recently found new favour among doctors and the general public. . . due to the publication of many works of scholarship on these subjects. . . so that, day by day, statistics are demonstrating that traditional, empirically-based notions were well-founded after all." Unfortunately, this research was done primarily in France and is not commonly available in the United States. However, his book, *The Practice of Aromatherapy*, is an excellent resource.

Dr. Valnet described an experiment performed by Professor C. Vallette and published by *C. R. Soc. Biologique* in 1945 as "Penetration Transcutanee des essences." High doses of essential oils applied to the skins of mice or rats caused immediate death; lower doses produced either depression or exaltation. Essential oils were found to pass quickly through the external layers of the skin and into the blood. Thyme and eucalyptus were absorbed in twenty to forty minutes; bergamot, lemon, and anise in forty to sixty minutes; citronella, pine, lavender, cinnamon, and geranium in sixty to seventy minutes, and the essences of mint, coriander and rue in approximately a hundred minutes.

Here are some of the properties that Dr. Valnet observed in regard to the 17 common oils that I describe in this book:

antiseptics (to inhibit growth of bacteria): lemon, lavender, eucalyptus

choleretics (to aid in the production and evacuation of bile): rosemary, lavender

to prevent formation of gallstones or urinary tract stones: juniper, lemon

antispasmodics and to calm the nerves: lavender

to stimulate the adrenal cortex: rosemary

tonics and to excite the anterior pituitary: lemon

to strengthen sexual faculties: ylang-ylang

to promote sweating: chamomile

to detoxify: lavender, rosemary

to prevent fermentation: lemon, juniper[22]

Researchers at the Pasteur Institute have discovered that oils of thyme, clove, mint, marjoram, pine, and oregano strongly inhibit the microbes that cause tuberculosis, cholera, and staphylococcal infections. In tests at Weber University, cinnamon oil proved more effective than ampicillin in inhibiting the growth of staphylococcal infections—without the bacteria acquiring resistance to the oil.[23]

In 1985, Dr. Jean C. Lapraz reported that he could not find bacteria or viruses that could live in the presence of the essential oils of cinnamon or oregano.[24]

John Tyndale discovered that essential oil molecules give off an infrared radiation that can be picked up by insects. The essential oils of patchouli, sandalwood, cloves, lavender, rose, lemon, thyme, rosemary, and anise seeds can absorb infrared rays. Infrared exposure improves circulation and opens blood vessels, bringing blood to the surface of the skin.[25]

Dr. Farag, head of biochemistry at the University of Cairo, documented the oxygenating molecular activity of essential oils, showing that some pure essential oils increase bodily oxygen by 21 percent (as compared to a 6 to 7 percent increase with herbs and vitamins, and a 9 percent increase with hydrogen peroxide). Many diseases, including cancer, cannot exist in the presence of oxygen. Oxygen creates better absorption of nutrients and a higher level of cellular regeneration. The small size of the molecules of the essential oils allows them to pass easily through the interstitial fluid easily, crossing the blood-brain barrier and entering the circulatory system rapidly.

According to Dr. Otto Warburg, Nobel Prize winner for cancer research, cancer occurs when the normal aerobic (in the presence of oxygen) respiration of the body's cells is replaced by an anaerobic (in the absence of oxygen) cell respiration. Hydrogen has a low Hertz frequency, so when cells are clogged with hydrogen (from eating hydrogenated oils in the form of margarine, shortening, and hydrogenated peanut butter, for example), essential oils can be introduced that vibrate at a rate far higher than the zero rate for processed foods. The excess oxygen generated by these oils can drive out the offending hydrogen.[26]

Herbalists Cathy Keville and Mindy Green explain, "Essential oils include muscle relaxants, digestive tonics, circulatory stimulants, and hormone precursors. Many repair injured cells; others carry away metabolic waste. In addition, a number of essential oils enhance immunity, working with the body to heal itself. They stimulate the production of phagocytes (white blood cells that attack invaders) and some are antitoxic. Many essential oils have been proven effective against fungi and yeast, parasites, and viruses. Others fight infection with amazing effectiveness, killing bacteria by disrupting their lifecycle.[27]

Essential oils have an electrical property called polarity that is expressed as positive or negative. The electro-positive warming oils, which are often red-orange in color (including oregano, thyme, clove and savory) lack an electron that they acquire from other cells, thereby producing heat. The electro-negative cooling oils including German chamomile, which is blue have an extra electron that they can donate. The neutral oils tend to be yellow or green, including lavender, clary sage, and Roman chamomile.

The chemical composition of an oil also gives clues about its electrical properties. There may be two hundred to eight hundred different chemical constituents in a single oil, and each constituent has a different effect on the body. Here some of the more common chemical types, along with some of their electrical properties:

aldehydes (electro-negative): anti-infectious, sedative, calming to the nervous system
eugenols: stimulating, antiseptic
ketones: stimulate cell regeneration and liquify mucus
phenols (electro-positive): antiseptic, kill viruses and bacteria
sesquiterpenes: anti-inflammatory, bring increased oxygen to the brain, stimulate the endocrine glands
terpene alcohols (electro-positive): antibacterial, diuretic, decongestant[28]

Dr. Valnet and Claude Reddet did research that was published as "Contribution a l'application pratique d'une nouvelle conception du terrain biologique" in *A.M.I.F.* April–May 1961. They studied the essential oils in terms of their pH value and electrical resistance.

The pH represents the acidity or alkalinity of a solution, in a range of 0 to 14.14, with pure water at 7.07. The lower the pH, the more acid the reaction; the higher the pH, the more alkaline. Resistance is the property of a solution to oppose the transmission of heat or electricity. Valnet explains, "The purer a solution, the less conductive it is to the transmission of electricity. The resistance of blood is on average 190 ohms/cm/cm$^2$ for a man, 220/230 for a woman." Natural essences usually have an acid pH value and a high resistance.

Valnet and Reddett found that essence of cloves has a resistance of 4000 ohms (20 times that of human blood), thyme has 3,300, lavender has 2,800, and mint has 3,000. A mixture of essences with strong bactericidal properties has a resistance of 17,000—much greater than the sum of its component essences— and a pH of 4.6. High acidity in this context prevents the rapid multiplication of microbes, and the high resistance discourages the diffusion of infections and toxins.[29]

## Frequencies of Essential Oils

During his work with plants, soil, and water in his agricultural projects, Bruce Tainio developed a machine called a BT3 Frequency Monitoring System (see Resources) that uses a highly sensitive sensor to measure the bio-electrical frequencies of essential oils and nutrients. Since there was no instrument at the time that could provide him with this information, he built the first BT3 Frequency Monitoring System, which has been modified and perfected over the years.

Tainio's website (http://www.tainio.com/ir/frqmonitor/faq. htm) explains that every atom in the universe has a specific vibratory motion. Each periodic motion has a frequency (the number of oscillations per second) that can be measured in Hertz.

I contacted Tainio to inquire about how his machine works. He explained that every element in the Periodic Table has a specific vibratory frequency. This has been documented in England. Most plants and creatures use enzymes to break down components, and each of these enzymes has a specific frequency.[30] The International Enzyme Commission published photos of these unique crystalline forms for every enzyme in the dried state. They can be seen in the back of a book called *Enzymes* by Malcolm Dixon and Edwin C. Webb.[31]

Since the elements and enzymes remain in the oils, the BT3 measures the composite frequency of the vibratory emissions in peak-to-peak electrical voltage. As a Hertzian wave is generated and travels out from its source, it transfers energy to the objects it passes through. The frequency monitor's sensor measures the nano voltage of that wave, using the predominant frequency in the megahertz range, filtering out the lower and higher ranges.

Measurements with Tainio's frequency monitoring system indicate that the average living plant is 20 to 22 MHz. The frequency of the fruit (after pollination) can be as high as 80 MHz.[32] Healthy nutritious plants always have a higher frequency than less healthy ones. Processed foods may be as low as zero, and whole foods may have frequencies up to 15 MHz. Dried herbs range from 12 to 22 MHz.[33]

Tainio found a way to measure a person's frequency by taking readings on various points of the body and averaging those numbers together. His measurements indicate that healthy human beings vibrate in the range of 62 to 68 MHz. Human cells start to change (mutate) when their frequency drops below 62 MHz.[34] When the acid-alkaline balance (which can be measured by pH papers) indicates an acidic condition, this will also be accompanied by a low frequency. Pathogens have a low frequency, and beneficial bacteria have a higher frequency. Negative thoughts will lower your body frequency in three seconds. Positive thoughts will bring your frequency up to optimum range in twenty-one seconds.[35]

I experienced this when I awoke after a very traumatic dream. On a hunch I used pH papers to measure the acid-alkaline balance of my saliva. The normal human range covered by my pH papers is from 5.5 to 8.0. My pH was at a low of 5.5. Ten minutes later I had an extremely happy thought. I felt so good that I had the impulse to measure my pH again. I had not eaten or had anything to drink, yet my pH had risen to 6.4!

According to measurements taken with Tainio's machine, when you have a cold or flu your vibratory rate goes down to 58 MHz. When candida is present you vibrate at 55 MHz; when Epstein-Barr virus is present you vibrate at 52 MHz; when cancer is present you vibrate at 42 MHz. When the death process begins, the frequency has been measured at 20 MHz.

Pure essential oils have strong frequencies, though adulterated oils may be as low as 0 MHz. Pure essential oils have been measured at 52 MHz for basil oil and 320 MHz for rose oil. Lavender was measured at 118 MHz, sandalwood at 96 MHz, and peppermint at 78 MHz. Measurements vary according to growing and harvesting conditions and purity of the oil. When you inhale an essential oil, there can be an immediate shift in your frequency level. Note that adulterated oils may actually lower your frequency level.[36]

According to scientist Dr. Royal Raymond Rife (1888–1971), every cell has its own vibratory resonance. A substance with a higher frequency will neutralize a disease with a lower frequency (the principle of entrainment—see Glossary).[37]

Essential oils create an environment in which low frequency diseases, harmful bacteria, viruses, and fungal diseases cannot survive. This means that using a deodorizing mouth rinse made of high-quality essential oils, for example, will both eliminate the immediate aesthetic problem of bad odor in the mouth, and it will remove the cause of the odor by fighting infections and neutralizing pathogens within the body. However, it is not a substitute for dental work.

Essential oils also influence the emotions, particularly oils in the high frequency ranges. Essential oils in the low frequencies have more effect on structural and physical changes, including cells, hormones, and bones, as well as viruses, bacteria, and fungi.[38]

## Author's Experience with Essential Oils

As a child, whenever I had a chest cold, my mother used a vaporizer with eucalyptus oil. It had the magical ability to loosen up phlegm. To this day, every drugstore in North America carries eucalyptus oil. There are also the effective cough drops that contain eucalyptus and camphor oils.

Essential oils are part of the art of herbology, and long before I heard the term aromatherapy I was using oils as part of my practice as an herbalist. Some of my most potent remedies involved the use of oils.

A popular remedy for all kinds of aches and pains (but not on mucous membranes) is a salve called Tiger Balm, which comes in a small round red vial from China. It contains camphor, as does Ben Gay, which comes in a tube, and is famous as a rub for chest colds. Tiger Balm also has a hefty amount of cajeput oil, mint oil, some menthol, and a little clove oil. It too can be rubbed full strength onto the chest and any place where there is pain.

One of my most effective early remedies was oil of bitter orange, derived from an inedible African orange. This is still my remedy of choice for systemic staph infections. Staphylococcus is a spherical-shaped bacterium that is very common in our environment and it is the infecting organism that causes boils. I've used this oil to clear up many serious cases of boils that would not respond even to antibiotics. (Take four drops or three drops for children in half cup of orange juice, three times a day until all symptoms are gone, and then for another three days. Boils usually clear up in one to three weeks, depending on the severity of the problem.)

Oil of bitter orange is also used for gum infections and sore throats (use a Q-Tip to paint it onto those areas, full strength). The inside of the mouth, gums, and tongue are associated with the second chakra, which is orange. The throat is associated with the third chakra, which is yellow, so it's not an exact match.

Peppermint and wintergreen oils are famous for settling the stomach and cleansing the breath, and are often used in breath mints and after dinner candies. As an herbalist, I frequently prepared peppermint tea for stomach complaints. Now I just rub a few drops of peppermint oil, neet (undiluted), over the painful area of the abdomen. For children, I dilute it in an equal amount of olive oil. Stomachaches, gas, and indigestion disappear almost instantly. Since most of the digestive organs are located in the third chakra, peppermint oil is associated with this chakra. Peppermint oil is also a reliable way to cure headaches when rubbed into the temples.

Another popular remedy during the 1960s was Essential Balm, which also comes from China in a round red vial. This brown salve contains a generous proportion of cinnamon and menthol, a medium amount of peppermint and eucalyptus, and a relatively small amount of clove, in a paraffin base. Probably because of the peppermint oil, it is excellent for headaches and stomachaches when rubbed, full strength, into the temples or abdomen.

Lavender oil is used in a wide variety of cosmetics, but you may not know how effective it is for alleviating pain (see the story below). I was introduced to this aspect of lavender oil when I went to a presentation about a multi-level company. The speaker showed us a tube of their cream and said that it had amazing powers for removing pain. He asked people in the audience to hold up their hands if they had any kind of pain. I was one of twenty people who raised their hands. I had sprained my finger.

The man passed the tube through the audience, and those of us who had pain rubbed a little bit of the cream into our painful parts. Fifteen minutes later he asked for a show of hands for how many people had experienced pain relief after using the cream. I was one of eighteen people who raised their hands. That impressed me. The only active ingredient in the cream that could account for this response was the lavender oil. I have since found that it is an important ingredient to add to massage oils, burn medications, and first aid ointments. Because of the violet color of its flowers and its ability to calm and soothe the nerves, lavender oil is associated with the higher chakras.

Another early herbal remedy was mullein oil. When I lived in the southwest in the early 1980s, I would go into the desert in the fall and gather tiny yellow flowers from the tall stalks of the mullein plant. I would pack these little flowers into a pint Mason jar and put on the lid and then place the jar on the hot roof of my house, where the sun caused the flowers to exude their oil. After a couple of weeks I would squeeze out the wilted flowers and harvest the precious oil. A whole pint would only yield a couple teaspoons, but if you had an earache, you only needed to put a few drops into the ear, and it would take the pain away. Mullein oil is available in many health food stores.

As an herbalist, I used to carry many containers full of dried herbs whenever I traveled or made house calls. Now I have a tiny satchel with small vials of essential oils that I use for virtually all the ailments I formerly needed herbs to cure.

## Practical Aspects of Aromatherapy

In this section we will look at how the essential oils are produced, and I will give instructions on how to use the oils for everyday purposes.

### How Essential Oils are Produced

Essential oils can be extracted from plants or trees—from the whole plant or from the seeds, flowers, petals, stems, roots, or bark. Two or more different oils may be taken from one plant. The orange tree, for example, yields orange oil from pressing the peel, petitgrain oil is distilled from the leaves and twigs, and neroli oil is produced from the blossoms.[39]

The quality of the oil depends upon many factors, including the process by which it was obtained, its state of maturity upon harvesting, and the location where it was grown. About 100 kilograms (220 pounds) of lavender plants, for example, are required to yield 2.9 kilograms (about six and a half pounds) of essential oil. So it is not surprising that oils are often adulterated with alcohol, fixed oils, essential oils of lower quality, and synthetic esters such as soap from animal fat or gelatin.[40]

An ancient method for extracting oils cited in the Ebers Papyrus was to strip cedar bark, grind it fairly fine, soak it with olive oil, wrap it in a wool cloth, and then set the cloth on fire. This would pull the essential cedar oil out of the bark into the olive oil. The cloth was then pressed and the oil extracted. In a refinement of this method, flower petals were placed in goose or goat fat, and then the oil was separated from the fat. This was the primitive beginning of a method now called **absolute**.[41]

**Distillation** is still considered the most economical method of extracting essential oils. Think of what happens when you cover a pot of water, bring it to a boil, and remove the lid. The water that drips from the lid has been lifted from the surface of the water in the pot through evaporation and has condensed as distilled water on the lid of the pan.

The word *volatile* is derived from the Latin *volare*, which means "to fly." The smallest molecules of the plant are the most volatile, and only these can evaporate. The **top note** in perfumery refers to these extremely small molecules. Oils that contain the heaviest and least volatile of these small molecules are called **base notes.**

In a still, steam enters a chamber and travels up through the plant material placed in the still. The volatile oil is driven out of the plant material and evaporates into the steam. It travels along a pipe, where it begins to cool. To hasten the cooling process, the pipe is immersed in a large vat of cold water, causing the oil to condense back into liquid. The oil tends to float to the top of the water (though some oils sink to the bottom) where it can be drawn off. The end product is pure, genuine, whole, and natural essential oil.[42]

Yet even then, there are degrees of purity. Gary Young, an aromatherapy authority, points out that, as the steam rises, the microfine membranes in the plant open, releasing the oil molecules. If the membranes are fractured, the molecular structure of the oil is altered. In ancient distillation, less than five pounds of pressure and low temperature were used to obtain the highest quality therapeutic oils. Marcel Espieu, the president of the Lavender Growers Association in southern France, claims that the best-quality oil is produced when the pressure is zero pounds.

Working with such extreme sensitivity during the extraction process produces oils that are particularly effective in healing. Young points out that these oils "must work on the areas in the brain that are connected to the limbic system, which affects emotional trauma release, appeases anxiety, and helps overcome depression. . . . High pressures and high temperatures seem to cause a harshness in the oil where even the oil pH and the electro-positive and electro-negative balance are greatly affected."

For example, Young's research has shown that the highest quality cypress oil requires twenty-four hours at a maximum of 245 degrees Fahrenheit at five pounds of pressure. Yet if it is distilled for less than twenty-two hours, eighteen to twenty of the primary constituents will be missing.[43] This may explain why French doctors who use high-quality therapeutic oils get positive results that may not be reproduced by American clinicians using lower grade oils.

For the highest-grade lavender oil, the lavender flowers should be harvested in full bloom, prior to the high heat of the day, and left in the field for two to three days. Then the oil should be distilled at low pressure and low temperature for one and one-half hours. Young explains:

> In the larger fields of the world during the distillation time, one can see chemical trucks hooked into the distillers, pumping solvents into the water already in the boiler. This increases the oil production by as much as 18 percent, and then they can say, 'Yes, it is steam distilled,' and 'No, we have not mixed chemicals with the oils, nor added propylene glycol to them.' However, when you put a chemical in the water and force this with steam into the plant, it causes a fracturing of the molecular structure of the oil. This alters its fragrance and constituents because you cannot separate the chemicals from the oil after it comes through the condenser.[44]

There is a hybrid lavender that produces lavendin oil that is highly antiseptic, but lacks many of the healing properties of true lavender. Most lavender oil sold in the United States is lavendin that has been cut with synthetic linolol acetate to improve the fragrance and then pumped up with propylene glycol or SD 40, an odorless solvent that increases the volume.[45]

**Aromatic water** is a by-product of the distillation process. Some of the larger molecules from the plant do dissolve in water, and these form the aromatic water, which has a different aroma than the essential oil of the same plant. Even today, many Arab women have tiny stills for making orange flower water for cooking and medicine. Unfortunately, almost all rose water found in pharmacies and commercial stores is made with synthetic substitutes.[46]

**Expression** is a form of extraction used exclusively with citrus fruits. The essential oil is simply cold-pressed out of the little sacs just under the surface of the rind. In the United States this is usually done in factories that produce fruit juice. Unfortunately, these companies spray their fruit with chemicals that are highly concentrated in the rinds of citrus.

**Solvent extraction** does not produce essential oils, but does produce some highly concentrated perfume materials. They always retain a small amount of the solvents, which may cause a reaction in sensitive people. There are three types of solvent extractions:

*Resinoids* are gumlike resins produced when an incision is made in certain trees or bushes. Solvents are used to extract the aromatic molecules from the resin. The solvents include hydrocarbons such as benzene or hexane, or alcohols. The solvents are filtered off and removed by distillation. When hydrocarbon solvents are used, the product is called a resinoid. When alcohol solvents are used, it is called an absolute resin.

*Concretes* also use hydrocarbons as a solvent, but instead of starting with a resin, the process uses the leaves, flowers, and roots of the plant. Most concretes are solid, waxlike substances. They are often used in food flavorings.

*Absolutes* also use alcohol as a solvent. The alcohol is then gently evaporated off to extract the aromatic molecules. Instead of starting with a resin or plant material, absolutes start with a concrete. This produces a thick, colored liquid. Absolutes and resins are not classed as essential oils. Jasmine absolute is popular, because there is no way to make essential oil of jasmine.[47]

**Hypercritical carbon dioxide (CO2) extraction** is a nonsolvent method of extracting the essence of the plant. Pressure is used to turn carbon dioxide gas into a safe, inert liquid solvent. Carbon dioxide is the gas that we normally exhale from our lungs. Unfortunately, the equipment to perform this procedure is presently so expensive that the cost of the products is very high. Two products are produced:

*Essential oils* or *CO2 selects* resemble classic steam distillate oils, but have no temperature degradation and are extremely pure.

*Totals* are extracts obtained at higher pressures. These resemble a classic hexane extract, without solvent residue. They are very much like the herb itself. They are thick and pasty and make excellent additions to creams, ointments, and soaps. They should not be used in a diffuser since they could clog the vents.[48]

## Precautions and Instructions for Using Essential Oils

Here are some basic precautions and instructions for using essential oils:

- Unless a carrier (see below) is indicated, essential oils may be applied **neet** (undiluted).

- When instructions call for a **carrier**, these are usually cold pressed vegetable, seed, and nut oils that carry the essential oil. Carriers are used in various proportions to add volume to the costly essential oils. Most vegetable oils bought in the grocery store are not cold-pressed and have less therapeutic benefit. Mineral oil is not used in aromatherapy because it attaches to your oil soluble vitamins (A, D, E, and K) and carries them out of your body.

  Jojoba is highly recommended because it is actually not an oil, but a liquid wax, so it will not go rancid. However, it penetrates skin rapidly, so it is not good to use as a massage oil. A good carrier for massage is almond oil, because it has a gentle aroma and is nourishing to the skin.

- Essential oils do not go rancid, but combinations that contain carrier oils (other than jojoba) do. To preserve combinations of oils in a carrier base, add a few drops of vitamin E oil and, if possible, store in the refrigerator. To warm the oils before using, place the unopened bottle in a pot of hot water and cover with a lid. Do not apply additional heat. Just let it sit for a few minutes.

- Wash your hands before and after using essential oils, and do not touch your fingers directly to the opening of the bottle.

This protects the oils from contamination and keeps you safe from inadvertently getting oils in your eyes and other mucous membranes and sensitive skin areas.

- Keep essential oils in green or brown glass bottles, to protect the oils from deterioration due to exposure to the sun. Store them in a cool dark place away from direct sunlight and heat. The oils will melt through plastic and rubber, so avoid transporting your oils in dropper bottles with rubber bulbs. Some bottles have plastic tops with a hole for single drops to pass through. These tops do not dissolve as readily. Keep bottles closed when not in use to prevent evaporation and accidental spillage.

- Keep essential oils out of the reach of children.

- If you have sensitive skin or if you are using oil on a child or using an oil for the first time, test it on a small area of skin before using it (especially if applying neet). Do not use essential oils such as menthol near the throat or neck of children under thirty months of age. If you are pregnant, or have high blood pressure, epilepsy, open wounds, diabetes, sensitive skin, or allergies, proceed carefully and consult an aromatherapist before using oils. The bottoms of the feet are usually a safe place to apply oils and they will spread throughout the body very rapidly. Remember that just sniffing can be effective.

- Remove contact lenses before working with oils, or be especially careful to wash your hands thoroughly before handling the lenses since the high phenol content in the essential oils may cause sticking problems or could damage the surface of the lenses.

- Never put essential oils in your eyes or ears. If you do so accidentally, do not flush with water (oil and water do not mix). Instead, dilute the oil by using a few drops of pure vegetable oil, such as olive oil, directly in the eyes. Then profuse flushing with warm water can be helpful.

- Citrus oils can make the skin photosensitive and may cause rashes or pigmentation changes when worn on an area that is exposed to direct sunlight, even three to four days after exposure. The high coumarin content of citrus oils allows the body to absorb more ultraviolet light. Rashes will usually disappear in a few days, but discoloration of the skin may last longer. If citrus oil is distilled, the coumarins will be removed.

- The following oils can be caustic to the skin and should be diluted with a carrier before application: citrus oils of bergamot, grapefruit, lime, lemon, tangerine, mandarin, and orange; conifer oils of birch, cedarwood, juniper, pine, and spruce; and spice oils of cinnamon, clove, basil, ginger, lemongrass, oregano, marjoram, nutmeg, pepper, and thyme. The most caustic oils are cinnamon, lemongrass, oregano, and thyme

- Do not eat or drink essential oils without first consulting an aromatherapist. Be sure to use only organic therapeutic grade oils, and never ingest absolutes, $CO_2$, or solvent-expressed or synthetic oils. Before ingesting, dilute essential oils in an oil-soluble liquid such as honey, milk, or olive oil, to facilitate assimilation and protect the delicate mucous membranes of the mouth and esophagus. If you are taking medication or if you are addicted to alcohol, tranquilizers, or any other substances, begin with half the recommended dosage of essential oils.[49]

## Common Uses of Essential Oils

I sometimes meet with skepticism from people who cannot understand how an inhaled substance can really affect the mind or the body, and I ask them to consider anaesthetics, nicotine or even glue-sniffing! Similarly, many find it hard to believe that oils absorbed through the skin can affect the whole organism, but even "orthodox" medicine is now coming around to the idea that some substances are even more effective when used transcutaneously.—*Patricia Davis*[50]

There are many ways to use essential oils. One of the best forms of preventive medicine is to get rid of all chemical household cleansers and poisons. One good resource for toxins related to common household cleansers is *The Cure for All Cancers* by Hulda Regehr Clark, N.D. Every household cleanser and poison can be replaced by remedies made with essential oils and herbs.

The following guidelines will help the beginner to understand how to use essential oils preventively and therapeutically.

**Sniff the Oil.** Open a bottle and sniff the oil. The microscopic molecules travel quickly when inhaled, easily penetrating the fatty layers of the skin. The body's response time to inhalation can be as rapid as one to three seconds.[51] It isn't necessary to consume the oil in any other way to receive its benefits. This is good to remember when using expensive oils.

**Using Oils with the Chakras.** First allow your client to smell the essential oil by holding the bottle under the nostrils, to be sure that it is agreeable. Then shake the oil onto your fingers. A dab of undiluted oil may be placed on the cheeks or temples so it can be smelled, and 1 to 6 drops may be applied directly to the area of the chakra. For the first chakra, apply to the tailbone area in back, but avoid mucous membranes. All other chakras can be applied to the front of the body. For reasons of modesty, allow your client to apply her own oils when that seems appropriate. For most sessions, it is good to use just one to three oils, so that their aromas can be individually appreciated.

**To Clean the Energy.** Pour ½ cup of warm water into a plant mister or spray bottle, and add 6 to 10 drops of angelica essential oil and G teaspoon sea salt or table salt. Hold your finger over the opening and shake vigorously to mix the oil and dissolve the salt. Angelica is excellent to spray in a room to remove bad energies. Do not combine with other oils when using it for this purpose.

**Massage Oil or Lotion.** Essential oils will travel directly through the cells of the skin, penetrating the fatty tissue layers into the interstitial fluids where they can enhance circulation.[52] Some nice massage combinations include lavender, rosemary, lemon, and ginger, separately or together. For deep penetration in painful areas use tropical basil and white birch. Use 10 to 20 drops of essential oil per fluid ounce of nut or vegetable oil or lotion. Use up to 10 percent jojoba if desired. Add the oils to the bottle, then roll the bottle back and forth between your hands to warm it (or place in hot water for a few minutes). Apply as needed, but avoid mucous membranes.

**Sensual Oils.** Essential oils are wonderful to enhance sexual pleasure, in massage lotion or in a diffuser, but should not be used near mucous membranes or in combination with rubber birth control devices. Lavender, neroli, ylang ylang, rose geranium, sandalwood, rose, and patchouli are pleasant and have aphrodisiac effects, if you like their odors.

**Bath Oils and Bath Salts.** Combine 1 to 6 drops of essential oil with an equal amount of vegetable oil. Run hot water in the tub, add the oils, and swish. To make bath salts, add 6 drops of essential oil per tablespoon of Kosher, Hawaiian, or Epsom salts. (There are 30 drops to ¼ teaspoon, and 8 tablespoons to ½ cup, so you would need one-quarter and ⅛ teaspoons of oil per one-half cup of salt.) Sprinkle about ½ cup of the bath salts directly under the hot water from the tap. Stir to dissolve, then add cool water until the bath water reaches a comfortable temperature. Pregnant women and children may want to avoid the caustic oils mentioned above. Lavender is great in the bath; it smells good and helps relieve aches and pains.

**Diffusers.** When oils are diffused into the air, they purify the air by increasing the atmospheric oxygen and boosting levels of beneficial ozone and negative ions, which inhibits the growth and reproduction of airborne pathogens.[53] One kind of diffuser sprays an ultra-fine mist that hangs in the air for hours. This type gives the longest lasting effects. Use 6 to 12 drops or more of essential oil in ¼ cup of a carrier. Another type of diffuser plugs directly into an electrical outlet, which generates heat that causes a piece of blotter paper to get so hot that the oil diffuses into the room. Place about 12 drops of essential oil onto the blotter paper. Diffusers may be disconnected every hour, for about 30 minutes before connecting again, because the nose ceases to smell aromas when they are constant. Lemon, peppermint, and pine are great for cleansing, and peppermint increases energy and concentration.

**Perfume.** For a pleasing aroma, dilute essential oils with an equal amount of carrier such as jojoba. Some favorites are lavender, gardenia, sandalwood, neroli, jasmine, and rose. Dab on the body as desired, avoiding mucus membranes.

**To Freshen the Air.** Pour ½ cup of warm water into a plant mister or spray bottle, and add 6 to 10 drops of essential oil and ¼ teaspoon sea salt or table salt. Hold your finger over the opening and shake vigorously to mix the oil and dissolve the salt. Keep a spray bottle over the toilet or other places where odor is a problem. All the citrus oils are effective and pleasant, as are lavender, pine, peppermint, and eucalyptus, separately or together. The solution may be harmful to clothing, eyes, or furniture, so spray away from people and fabric.

**Closet Fresheners and Insect Repellents.** Mothballs and camphor cakes are made with camphor oil. If you don't care for this smell, try putting a few drops of essential oil of clove, lavender, or cedarwood on a strip of cloth or a cotton ball in the closet. Refresh as needed.[54]

**Removing or Preventing Fleas.** Purchase or make a cloth collar for your pet's neck. Apply 1 drop of essential oil for a cat and 3 to 4 drops for a larger dog, every 3 days during flea season (when you see your pet scratching). Begin with 60 percent carrier oil (not jojoba) and 15 percent citronella oil, and then fill the remaining bottle with 2 or 3 of the following: rosemary, lavender, eucalyptus, lemon, or cedar.

**Removing Odors.** Add 5 to 10 drops of essential oil to your laundry load, or put onto a handkerchief and add it to the dryer. Soak noxious-smelling compost and bleach and other containers with hot water and a few drops of essential oil. Lemon oil is excellent. Lavender and pine are also good.

## Healing with Essential Oils

Fragrant oil brings joy to the heart
and a friend's support is as pleasant as perfume.
—*Proverbs 27:9*

**Emotional Healing.** Valerie Worwood, author of *The Fragrant Mind*, recommends the following oils for the corresponding emotional symptoms (I have condensed her list to the seventeen oils mentioned in this book.)

> To combat fear: frankincense, Roman chamomile, sandalwood
> To assuage guilt: jasmine, rose otto
> To alleviate feelings of unworthiness: frankincense, geranium, neroli, sandalwood, ylang ylang
> To facilitate letting go: frankincense, juniper, lemon
> To help receive love: lavender, neroli, Roman chamomile, rose otto, orange[55]

**Emotional Release.** Human beings give off pheromones and other chemicals when fearful and under stress. To cleanse the air when emotions are high, spray with a combination of angelica and lavender. This is also a good combination to use after doing emotional release work, or when you come into a room where the energy does not feel clean.[56]

**Auric Healing.** Harry Oldfield, an early British pioneer in Kirlian photograph (see Glossary) and a recipient of diplomas in homeopathy, biology, and physics, developed a method of viewing the human energy field, called Polycontrast Interface Photography (PIP). Through these photos one can witness essential oils being placed in the palm of a person's hand as his or her aura gets brighter and wider than the fields of control subjects in which no oils are used.[57] Presumably, when the aura is brighter and wider, the chakras are more open, and energy flows more freely through the body, mind, and spirit.

## Correlating the Oils with the Chakras

The following oils are arranged according to the chakras where I most commonly use them. These are just guidelines. Any essential oil may be used at any part of the body, provided that the cautions mentioned earlier are observed.

**First Chakra.** Aromas that have aphrodisiac properties are associated with the first and second chakras. If you want an aphrodisiac, be sure the aroma is pleasing to both parties. For the first chakra, I recommend the musky animalistic odors (which are not enjoyed by all), and for the second, the more subtle aromas. Also for the first chakra, I use oils that give a sense of grounding and connecting with the earth.

*Patchouli* is a thick dark yellowish brown oil with a greenish tinge. It is musty and pungent and—for those who like its distinctive odor—it has an aphrodisiac affect. It can be used as a perfume, though you may want to dilute it with up to ten parts carrier oil, such as almond oil. Patchouli is a stimulant and antidepressant that is commonly used in China, Japan, and Malaysia. It is useful for cracked skin, cracked heels, and athlete's foot (the feet are associated with the first chakra).

*Geranium* and particularly *rose geranium* are light green and vaguely recall the scent of rose oil. They can be used as a perfume by placing a few drops behind the ears. Both oils stimulate the adrenal cortex, which governs the balance of hormones, including male and female sex hormones. They are helpful for premenstrual tension and menopause, and are also used for fluid retention, which often occurs premenstrually.

**Second Chakra.** The aromatic oils for the first and second chakras are fairly interchangeable.

*Jasmine* is a dark, viscous oil with a heavy, almost animalistic quality. The white flowers must be gathered at night, when their aroma is strongest. High-quality jasmine oil is expensive, but only a tiny amount is needed and can be mixed with a carrier oil such as jojoba, or it can simply be inhaled. Massage jasmine oil on the abdomen and lower back during childbirth to relieve pain and strengthen contractions, and it can be used for postnatal depression. Jasmine strengthens the male sex organs and helps reduce an enlarged prostate. Its aphrodisiac properties may be helpful with both impotence and frigidity.

*Sandalwood* is a small evergreen parasitic tree that grows in India, Australia, and Hawaii. The oil is yellowish to deep brown and is extremely thick and viscous. A powerful antiseptic, it is used to treat infections of the urinary tract and gonorrhea. It is helpful for oily skin and acne and dry skin, and is excellent in after-shave lotions for barber's itch (the cheeks correspond to the second chakra). Sandalwood is also an effective aphrodisiac.

*Neroli* is a thick, deep brown oil derived from the flowers of orange trees. The bittersweet scent is best diluted in a carrier base. It is antidepressant, antiseptic, antispasmodic, and aphrodisiac. As a gentle sedative, it alleviates states of anxiety, including those associated with sexual performance, stage fright, and taking exams. Neroli helps promote sleep when added to a bath before bedtime. Because it stimulates growth of new skin cells, it is useful to prevent or heal scar tissue. Neroli is good for dry and sensitive skin. It is used to alleviate spasm of the smooth muscle, so rub it onto the abdomen for diarrhea and abdominal spasms.

**Third Chakra.** The digestive organs, the nerves, and the mind are associated with the third chakra. Essential oils are excellent for calming the nerves, soothing the digestion, and stimulating the mind, used internally and externally.

*Peppermint oil,* used in candy and various medications, is famous for settling the stomach and freshening the breath. The throat corresponds to the third chakra. Peppermint has a beneficial effect on the stomach, liver, and intestines. You can massage the stomach with peppermint oil with an equal amount of a carrier base as an antispasmodic for colic, indigestion, vomiting, and stomach flu. For headaches, a few drops are rubbed into the temples.

*Roman chamomile* oil is produced from a yellow flower. It is soothing, calming, and anti-inflammatory. Add a few drops to massage oil or apply neet to the abdominal area for internal inflammatory conditions such as colitis, gastritis, and chronic diarrhea. Add a few drops to a warm bath to alleviate stress or tension.

*Lemon oil* relieves anxiety and depression, and combats fatigue and lack of energy. Add a few drops to warm massage oil and apply to the back in light, gentle strokes. Use in a diffuser for stimulating the memory and for mental alertness. To relieve vomiting, put a couple drops on a tissue and inhale. For diarrhea, put a few drops in massage oil and gently massage the lower abdomen and lower back, then inhale from the hands with several slow deep breaths.

**Fourth Chakra.** The following oils are good for the heart and lungs.

*Ylang ylang* (pronounced E-Lang) comes from pink, mauve, and yellow flowers of a small tropical tree. The oil varies from almost colorless to pale yellow, and the aroma is extremely heavy and sweet. It is used to slow down overrapid breathing (hyperpnea) and overrapid heartbeat (tachycardia), and helps alleviate conditions of shock, anger, and high blood pressure. Ylang ylang is antidepressant, sedative, and aphrodisiac, as it helps reduce the anxiety associated with sexual performance. It also helps balance the male and female energies. Too much can cause nausea and/or headache.

*Rose oil* is not distilled, but is produced by enfleurage, which requires a huge quantity of rose petals. Consequently, the cost is very high, but only a tiny amount is needed. This deep reddish brown or greenish orange oil is a gentle but potent antidepressant and is especially comforting for those who are grieving. Rose water has similar uses, and since it is produced by distillation, it is far less expensive.

**Fifth chakra.** These oils correlate with the fifth chakra because of their blue flowers, or blue oil, or because they are beneficial for the ears (the part of the head that relates to the fifth chakra).

*German (blue) chamomile* oil is produced from a daisylike yellow and white flower. The soothing, calming, and anti-inflammatory properties of German chamomile are due to azulene, the active principle. When the oil is highly distilled, the azulene causes it to turn blue. Add a few drops to a carrier oil and apply directly to the skin for reddened skin conditions including rashes and inflammations. Add a few drops to a warm bath to alleviate stress or tension. It is also soothing, calming, and antidepressant. Just dab a couple of drops, undiluted, on the face. Rub it in to remove the blue color. For calming babies, add a few drops to massage oil or use drops diluted in oil for the bath. For earache, rub around the ear. Since the chamomile flower is yellow, this oil is also good for the third chakra. Be aware that this oil can stain clothing.

*Eucalyptus* oil, used for cooling the body, helps reduce fevers. During hot days, eucalyptus trees seem to give off a blue haze. Eucalyptus oil may be used in a hot or cold vaporizer to ease a tight, dry cough. Add ¼ teaspoon to ¼ cup warm water to use in gargles. Add a few drops to massage oil to relieve muscular aches and pains and reduce inflammation and fever.

**Sixth Chakra.** These oils relate to the mind, the head, and the nervous system.

*Rosemary* oil, derived from a pinelike evergreen, helps balance body and mind. It awakens the higher intuition, clears the mind, and strengthens the memory. Rosemary oil relieves headaches, migraines, and fatigue. Rub neet into the third eye or the temples. By adding about 10 drops to a quart of warm water, it makes the hair shiny and eliminates dandruff when used in a rinse.

*Juniper* oil is made from the ripe purple berries of the juniper bush. The oil helps overcome anxiety, insomnia, and mental fatigue when rubbed into the third eye. Add a few drops to your shampoo to counteract greasy hair and dandruff. Add a few drops to massage oil and rub over the kidney region to strengthen the kidneys and relieve fluid retention.

**Seventh Chakra.** These oils are also good for the head and nerves, and help create a spiritual atmosphere.

*Lavender* oil is recommended for all ailments of the head, brain, and nerves. Several drops may be added safely to the bath or to massage oil or used neet on the skin as perfume. Rub the oil neet into the solar plexus to calm spasms. Dab it onto your face or diffuse into the room for insomnia, infections, allergies, fainting, headaches, migraines, influenza, hysteria, and tension.

*Frankincense* oil comes from a resin with a somewhat camphorous, penetrating aroma. It has the ability to slow and deepen the breath, which contributes to feelings of calmness, which in turn is conducive to meditation. Frankincense is used in massage and bath oils for respiratory infections, chronic bronchitis, and asthma, and for those who have had strokes. Frankincense helps those who tend to dwell too much on their past.

PART 6

# Healing with Crystals

No ASPECT OF HEALING HAS BEEN AS MALIGNED AND MISUNDER-
stood as healing with crystals. Some people call this kind of healing "woo woo." For others, the idea that crystals have special
healing powers is whimsical at best and downright ridiculous at
worst. Yet there seems to be no contradiction in their minds in
knowing that all of modern technology—including digital clocks,
computers, CDs, and lasers—is dependent upon crystals.

In this section, I will explain how crystals are used in modern
technology. As you come to understand the remarkable powers of
crystals, you will begin to appreciate how these same powers relate
to your body and your consciousness.

Marcel Vogel (1917–1991) was a research scientist for IBM for
twenty-seven years. He received numerous patents for his inventions including the magnetic coating for the twenty-four-inch hard
disc drive systems still in use. He specialized in liquid crystal systems. As a child he had a near-death experience in which he experienced an overwhelming sense of light and love that would
influence his work in later years.

In 1969, he read about human-plant communication, and
though he was skeptical, he tried to duplicate these strange experiments that seemed to indicate that plants respond to thought. He
used split-leaf philodendrons connected to a Wheatstone bridge
(see Glossary) to compare a known resistance to an unknown
resistance. He found that when he pulsed his breath through his
nostrils, while holding a thought in his mind, the plant responded
dramatically. He said, "I learned that there is energy connected
with thought. Thought can be pulsed and the energy connected

with it becomes coherent and has a laser-like power."[1] The details of his work with plants are described in *The Secret Life of Plants* by Peter Tompkins and Christopher Bird and *Psychic Exploration: A Challenge to Science* edited by Edgar Mitchell.

In another experiment in 1974, Vogel wondered if it was possible to project thought into crystalline form. He believed that the purest force and the greatest cohering agent is love. He compared it to gravity, which attracts and coheres at every level of existence. To test his theory, he grew a crystal in his lab and for one full hour he projected unconditional love and the image of Mother Mary toward that crystal. He told me this story during a visit to San Jose in 1989, and showed me the crystal; it did have some resemblance to the robed figure of the Madonna.

In more recent times, Japanese researcher Masaru Emoto (see the Introduction on page xi) showed in his book, *The Message from Water*, how crystal patterns formed in frozen drops of water. The water crystals seem to respond to emotions, words, music, and essential oils. In one experiment, Emoto wrote *thank you* on a bottle of water and left it overnight, and by the next morning a strong symmetrical crystal pattern formed. He wrote *you fool* on a bottle of water and left it overnight, and by the next morning it formed a whirling pattern with a central explosion of energy.

Your body is 70 percent water. If Emoto's experiments are accurate, the water in your body imprints constantly from your environment. You absorb the emotions of people who are in your daily environment. You absorb the frequencies of music and other sounds and aromas in your environment. You also absorb the energies of crystals placed on your body. Researchers in England did an experiment similar to Emoto's with an amethyst crystal, and the frozen ice revealed the pattern of tiny amethysts.

As humans we like to believe that we have dominion over all the "lesser" kingdoms—yet, in some sense, the opposite is true. No other life form has such a delicate, unstable, easily influenced energy field. Every life form that interacts with you leaves its mark upon you.

So perhaps this section is not just about using crystals for healing. Perhaps it is more about the crystal that you are than the crystals that you use. It is about that mysterious phenomenon called consciousness, and another intangible called love, and the amazing way that we are connected to the mineral kingdom and the plant kingdom and All That Is.

## Cultural and Spiritual Uses of Crystals

The Hopi Indians of Arizona had a deep understanding of chakras and Vibrational Healing, including healing with crystals, as illustrated in the following story:

> The First People knew no sickness. Not until evil entered the world did persons get sick in the body or head. It was then that a medicine man, knowing how man was constructed, could tell what was wrong with a person by examining these centers. First he laid his hands on them: the top of the head, above the eyes, the throat, the chest, the belly. The hands of the medicine man were seer instruments; they could feel the vibrations from each center and tell him in which life ran strongest or weakest. Sometimes the trouble was just a bellyache from uncooked food or a cold in the head. But other times it came "from outside," drawn by the person's own evil thoughts, or from those of a Two Hearts. In this case the medicine man took out from his medicine pouch a small crystal about an inch and a half across, held it in the sun to get it in working order, and then looked through it at each of the centers. In this manner he could see what caused the trouble and often the very face of the Two Hearts person who had caused the illness. There was nothing magical about the crystal, medicine men always said. An ordinary person could see nothing when he looked through it; the crystal merely objectified the vision of the center which controlled his eyes and which the medicine man had developed for this very purpose...[2]

To this day, Hawaiians have a sacred relationship with the rocks. I had the privilege of attending the annual festival of Hawaiian hula troops (*Molokai Ka Hula Piko*) in celebration of the birth of hula on the little island of Molokai in May of 1997, where *kumu hula* (hula teacher) John Kaimikaua gave a series of talks. John comes from a long lineage of *Kahunas (*priests). He told us that the Hawaiian people used stones as archives, to store their *mana* (energy). Spherical rocks are considered sacred in Hawaii, just as they are in India. John said the deities sometimes used these boulders as resting places. It is also believed that the gods put their *ina*—their knowledge of healing—into certain boulders, which are called *pohaku*. When *Kahunas* need to know how to heal they sit with these revered stones and tune into their wisdom.[3]

There is a tradition among Hawaiians (and Native Americans and Australian Aborigines) of asking permission before picking a flower or taking a rock. My hula teacher, Raylene Ha'alelea Kawaiae'a, explains that in the Hawaiian tradition you always talk to the rocks and tell them what you intend to use them for, and then ask if they are willing to come. If they agree, then you must be conscientious to use all of them for the purpose that you stated. We do this when we go to the streambed to gather the flat, thin *ili ili* stones that are used as musical instruments for certain hula dances. Two *ili ili* are held in each hand and clicked together, like Spanish castanets. We do the same when we gather branches from the vy-vee tree, to use in the stick dance, or large leaves from the ti plant, to weave leis (circles of flowers or leaves). These are living traditions that have been passed along throughout the history of these people.

The old Hawaiians built their *heiaus* (temples) on a foundation of lava rocks. Before a temple could be built, the *kahuna* had to ask and receive permission from the rocks. King Kamehameha III (1758–1819) wanted to build a *heiau* at his birthplace. But when they were asked, the rocks in that area did not want to be used for that purpose. The kahunas asked the rocks in neighboring areas, and they too refused. Finally they went about twenty miles down the road, where the rocks gave their permission to be used for the *heiau*. King Kamehameha had his soldiers form a human chain between the two places, and they passed the rocks down the line.

Egyptian pyramids and tombs were full of lapis and malachite. Topaz symbolized Ra, the Sun God. Jade amulets were found in profusion in the tombs and burial chambers of Egypt, since they were believed to have the power to guide souls in the afterworld.

Lapis was frequently carved into the likeness of an eye, then ornamented with gold, as an amulet of great power. It represented the truth, and only Egyptian priests and royalty were permitted to wear such a gem around their necks. Malachite was ground into a fine eye powder and used by royalty and priests to stimulate clear vision and insight. Bloodstone was powdered and mixed with honey and egg white to cure tumors and stop hemorrhaging.

The Chinese traditionally attribute extensive healing powers to jade, including a long life and a peaceful death. Asians believed that emerald would strengthen memory, increase intelligence, and give the owner the power to foretell future events.

Amethyst was known as the stone of royalty and the Bishop's Stone. It is still worn on the fourth finger of the right hand of a Catholic bishop to symbolize ecclesiastical dignity and authority.[4]

In 1609, Anselmus De Boot, court physician to Rudolph II of Germany, wrote that angels could enter precious stones and guard men from dangers. He wrote, "That gems or stones, when applied to the body, exert an action upon it, is so well proven by the experience of many persons that any one who doubts this must be called over-bold. We have proof of this power in the carnelian, the hematite, and the jasper, all of which, when applied, check hemorrhage."[5]

In England in 1913, after extensive research led to the publication of his book *The Curious Lore of Precious Stones*, George Frederick Kunz concluded, "For the Middle Ages and even down to the seventeenth century, the talismanic virtues of precious stones were believed in by high and low, by princes and peasants, by the learned as well as by the ignorant."[6] He notes that there was also a prevailing belief that "the very substance of certain stones was liable to modification by the condition of health or even by the thoughts of the wearer. In case of sickness or approaching death the lustre of the stones was dimmed, or else their bright colors were darkened, and unfaithfulness or perjury produced similar phenomena."[7]

## Science of Crystals

Ancient Greeks found clear quartz crystals in the Alps and thought they were ice that was frozen so hard it would never melt. So they gave the find their word for ice, *krystallos*. As knowledge of minerals and chemistry grew, the word was applied to all minerals that have precise geometrical shapes. With the discovery of the microscope, it was found that even common table salt has a precise geometric shape, with flat faces at definite angles to one another.

In 1660, Nicolaus Steno found that all quartz crystals have certain angles in common. He reasoned that these angles are maintained by accumulating new layers of particles on the exterior rather than through internal growth, as observed in plants and animals.[8] Crystals are now defined as being enclosed by symmetrically arranged plane surfaces that intersect at definite and characteristic angles.[9]

The atomic arrangement of crystals was determined in 1912 with the invention of X-ray crystallography, the study of the symmetries of atomic structure within crystals. We now know that the atoms of crystals are arranged in fixed, regularly repeating patterns.[10] This includes red garnet, smoky quartz, citrine, rose quartz, watermelon tourmaline, clear quartz crystal, fluorite, and amethyst. Technically, all metals are crystals. Rocks, trees, and bones are also crystals. Glass, however, is not a crystal because its molecular structure lacks a fixed, regularly repeating structure. Volcanic obsidian cools too quickly to allow molecules to move into their natural crystalline structure.[11] Although it's technically not a crystal, volcanic rock is important for healing.

There are seven divisions that make up the classification of crystal systems based on the crystalline lattice structures. These are the triclinic, monoclinic, orthorhombic, tetragonal, hexagonal, cubic, and trigonal systems.

Because crystals are extremely orderly, they have the lowest possible state of entropy (a state of maximum homogeneity in which all matter is at a uniform temperature). The crystalline structure is highly responsive to heat, light, pressure, sound, electricity, and other forms of electromagnetic energy.

When mechanical pressure is applied to quartz crystals, they respond by emitting a spark that gives off a measurable electrical voltage. This is called the piezoelectric effect (pronounced *pie-ee'-zo*). The oscillations of this charge are so regular and precise that they can be used to measure bits of time, which is why they are the primary component of most timepieces.

Scientists grow specific crystals from silicon dioxide for a wide variety of different applications. By adding other elements during the formative stage, it is possible to produce highly sensitized crystals for electrical conductivity, optical activity, and thermal conductivity. This is called doppling.

Each slice or plate of quartz has its own natural resonant frequency, depending upon its exact size and thickness. When an alternating current is passed through the plate, the charge will oscillate at a given numbers of cycles per second, according to the resonant frequency of the crystal. If the charge is strong enough it will activate mechanical movement. This is the basis for silicon wafers or chips that are primary components used in electronic devices and solar technologies.[12]

Storage is one of the numerous scientific uses of crystals. Oak Ridge National Laboratories in Tennessee has been storing thousands of three-dimensional images in single crystals. Just rotating the crystal slightly creates new storage possibilities. Phillips Research Labs of Hamburg, Germany recorded a demonstration holographic movie in a lithium niobate crystal. The potential for archival storage is tremendous.[13]

In the field of communications, a tiny gallium arsenide crystal has been used to display information via light-emitting diodes (LEDs). Liquid crystal displays (LCDs) are seen on laptop computers, clocks, inexpensive temperature-biofeedback devices, and miniature color TV sets.[14] Liquid crystal is neither a solid nor a liquid because its molecules tend to maintain their orientation, like those in a solid, but also move around to different positions, like those in a liquid. The predictable way that liquid crystal reacts to the passage of electrical current makes it possible to control the passage of light, which makes it well suited for producing LCDs.[15]

Normally X-rays pass through most things with minimal scattering or absorption. Crystals, however, scatter the rays, making symmetrical patterns of bright spots, reflecting the rays at specific angles. When these angles are analyzed, they reveal the arrangement of planes and the distances between them. This allows a technician to observe the structure of biological substances, including DNA (from which genes are made) and myoglobin (an oxygen carrier in the human body).[16]

When one considers all of these uses of crystals, it no longer seems far-fetched to imagine that crystals may also be able to respond to the thought waves of consciousness.

Scientist Marcel Vogel stated that the crystal is a neutral object with an inner structure that is in perfect balance. "When it's cut to the proper form and when the human mind enters into relationship with its structural perfection, the crystal emits a vibration which extends and amplifies the powers of the user's mind." Vogel explained that the crystal worked like a laser to radiate energy in a coherent and concentrated form that could be projected into objects or people.[17]

William A. Tiller, Ph.D., is a crystallographer, at the Department of Material Sciences and Engineering at Stanford University, describes the geometrical pattern of frequencies:

We live in an ocean of frequencies as a fish lives in the water. The fish is unaware of the many possibilities of the medium in which he moves. So Man has been totally unaware of the possibilities of the vast ocean of frequencies in which he lives. The many energy frequencies move in geometrical patterns. When the geometrical patterns are altered, their manifestation is altered. Crystals are those substances which alter the geometrical pattern of frequencies. We must realize that these frequency patterns are more or less stable, but that crystals, because of their strength of geometrical pattern, can modify and reform the frequency pattern. In doing so, energy can be released and directed to Man's purposes. . . . The crystalline forms are the key patterns for the way the energies are built in the universe; and the key to unlocking energy in a constructive way. [18]

## Author's Experience with the Stones

I was first introduced to crystals for healing in 1984. That was in the era before personal computers, when the electric typewriter was rapidly replacing the old manual typewriter. I found it exhausting to sit in front of an electric typewriter for hours at a time. When I mentioned this to a friend, she asked, "Have you tried using an amethyst?"

The only thing I knew about amethysts was that they were purple stones that were supposed to be the birthstone for Aquarius, my astrological sign. I couldn't fathom the connection between amethysts and typewriters. But she showed me a book that said amethysts were good for protection. I couldn't imagine that it would help me with my typewriter, but she took me to a local rock shop and showed me an amethyst pendant that I liked. It was reasonably priced, and I was willing to try it.

I was working then as an herbalist, having written three books about herbal remedies. Most people in the early 1980s were highly skeptical about the healing power of herbs, and I did not wish to be equally as prejudiced about the healing power of rocks. Maybe it was wishful thinking, but the amethyst did seem to help.

I kept the pendant in my purse and shortly thereafter went to my first psychic fair. When I walked into the huge building, I felt assaulted by good energy and terrible energy. I was about to leave when I thought that perhaps the amethyst could protect me. I took out my little pendant and put it around my neck. Suddenly it seemed as if the negative energy was being blocked out. Today I have a necklace with a large amethyst crystal that I wear whenever I'm in a situation where I need protection. It feels extremely effective.

The word amethyst means "without drunkenness." This purple crystal is reputed to prevent negative side effects from alcohol. There is a story about a king who had a goblet carved out of amethyst, which he used to drink his fellow statesmen under the table. I had stopped drinking alcohol because it made me feel sleepy. So I purchased a little tumbled amethyst and dropped it into the bottom of my wineglass and, sure enough, I was able to drink with less drowsiness.

In the early 1990s, I moved to the Kootenay Mountains in the interior of British Columbia. A friend took me to a stream in an untouched forest of giant old-growth trees where the paths were overgrown. We were completely alone. We each sat down to meditate on a boulder on either side of the stream. I told her that I wanted to enter into the consciousness of the boulder. She agreed and we sat in silence for a long time.

Entering into a deep state of meditation, I felt my metabolism slowing down. My heart beat slowed, my breaths came slowly if at all, and I had a profound sense of expansion, particularly in my head. My whole being was going slower . . . . and slower . . . . and slower . . . . until my consciousness merged with the consciousness of the old-growth trees. They seemed to be speaking to me telepathically. "You humans think you are so special, just because you can move around! We have seen your kind come and go, come and go. You are so tiny, and your lives are so short."

Then I felt my metabolism slowing down even more. The tree consciousness fell away, and my heart was barely beating as my awareness sank down . . . . down . . . . down . . . . and I became one with the boulder beneath me. I felt so ancient! So all-encompassing. I had a sense that the rocks held the essence of place-ness. Yet when I felt myself as a rock, I did not feel solid. I felt airy. And still. Very, very still. Quiet. Centered.

I could feel my deep connection with other rocks along the streambed, many of which had broken off from me. I could feel both our separateness and our connectedness. The unity I felt with these other rocks existed beyond space and time, in another dimension. The boulder told me that when a rock breaks off from the mother rock, it remains in communication with her. I was told that it was good to gather rocks that come from the same mother, so that when a member of your community goes away, you can give him or her "a piece of the rock," to help maintain your connection with each other.

A few months later, I was driving through the Kootenay Mountains, past a rock face that always felt powerful to me. A hunk of rock had broken off from the rock face and fallen on the road, crumbling into many pieces. I stopped my car and went to gather some of these precious rocks. I was well rewarded for my efforts, because they were filled with red garnets. To this day, my family and friends have pieces of this rock.

I remembered this concept when I read about a phenomenon in quantum physics: in certain instances, when you do something to one of two subatomic particles, the action will affect the other, whether they are ten feet or ten billion miles apart. Yet physicists cannot explain how these signals are sent back and forth, because the signals have to travel faster than the speed of light, and according to Einstein, nothing can travel faster than the speed of light.[19]

I believe that rock consciousness exists outside time and space, perhaps in a parallel reality. My mother and I had instantaneous telepathic communication at times, and I believe that our communication was akin to rock consciousness. I believe that when I travel out-of-body (during past-life regressions, for example), I step outside the space-time continuum and then reenter it at a different location.

The experience of moving outside time was well documented in 1892 when Albert von st. Gallen Heim published a collection of accounts by mountain climbers who had fallen in the Alps and by others who had similar experiences. His book, *Remarks on Fatal Falls*, was translated into English in 1972.[20]

During their life-threatening falls, all the climbers experienced a significant enhancement of mental activity and clarity as they observed their situation and considered the possible outcome of events. Time became greatly expanded, and individuals acted with lightning speed and accurate reality testing. They each reported seeing their entire life in review, a process that would normally take many hours but happened in just a matter of seconds.[21]

I went to northeastern California to visit my friend, Swami Tayumanavar. When he was a child, his grandmother's best friend was a Native American medicine woman, so he was well-versed in

Indian lore. He and I were driving through the desert when he pointed to a hill and casually mentioned that the Indians believed that the hill held the essence of rock consciousness.

"Then let's stop!" I cried out, and he willingly pulled over to the side of the road. We trudged over to a couple of boulders that had fallen down from the hill. "Let's sit on these boulders," I suggested. "If they hold crystal consciousness, maybe they can help me understand why the crystals are so powerful."

So we each sat on a boulder at the foot of the hill in the middle of the desert, and, once again, I felt my metabolism slow down as I merged with the consciousness of the boulder. When I felt connected, I asked my question. To my amazement, I received a coherent answer: "After the Great Flood, remember that Yahweh was so distressed with what he had done that he vowed never to do that again. To seal his covenant with his people, he put his bow in the sky, to remind him of his promise. So the rainbow is the manifestation of God's emotions. When you bring the rainbow down to earth, you have the multicolored minerals. So the healing stones are hunks of God's emotions."

I was amazed. Now I understood why my first client who was grieving over the loss of her boyfriend, but who could not cry, broke out crying when I placed the rose quartz on her heart. Rose quartz is reputed to contain the essence of unconditional love. You might say that it holds the essence of the feminine aspect of God's loving energy.

How blessed we are by the presence of these jewels in our lives. As Swami Tayumanavar says, "The inner teachings of the Eastern priesthoods tell us that crystals appear in the spiritual realms much as they do in the physical world, so they can be used by angelic intelligences to carry vibrations from one plane of existence to another."

## Using the Stones

Each healing stone has a unique energy, just as you have your own unique energy. Each category of stones also has a unique energy, much as your family has its own characteristics. Think of your uncle. How do you feel about him? How would you describe him? Do your other siblings experience him exactly the way you do? Does your mother? Do your friends? Your perception of your uncle is a reflection of how your energy and personality interact with his. Your sister may see him completely differently. You may think he is funny, and she may think he is corny.

It is the same with the stones. I may experience obsidian, a black volcanic rock, as being grounding, and you may experience it as being uplifting. There is no way to be wrong about your perceptions. If it is uplifting to you; that is your truth. Use it that way. Don't let anyone tell you otherwise. It would be a shame, for example, if you stopped laughing at your uncle's jokes, just because your sister doesn't like them.

You will find contradictory information in different books about the qualities of the crystals. Yet there is also a great deal of agreement—just as there is some degree of consensus in a given community about whether a particular woman is good-hearted and generous or whether she is stingy and selfish.

For this reason, I am reluctant to assign qualities to the stones. But when you are learning to use them, unless you are extremely intuitive and able to trust your intuition, it may be difficult to tune in to them. So you can begin with my descriptions. Ideally, take time to get your own readings. In fact, if you have two pieces of obsidian, they may share some qualities, but each may have its unique characteristics (especially if they are have different sizes and shapes and if they were mined in different locations).

Bear in mind when you are working with a friend or client that he may not experience the energy of a given stone the same way you do. So it is always good to pause for a minute after placing a stone on his body, and ask, "How does that feel?" Tell him he can move the stone around any way he wants. Reassure him that he may not feel anything, but the stone is still doing its work. If he says that it feels heavy (note that very large stones can feel light, and small stones can feel heavy), or disturbing, offer to remove the stone and try another one.

## Reading a Stone

Approach a new crystal like a newborn baby. When I see a new baby, the first thing I do is look in her eyes. Then I may I look at her hair, ears, fingers, and toes. I like to look at a crystal with the same wonder, curiosity, and appreciation.

When you consider a stone think about its signature. In herbalism, the signature of plants is a phenomenon in which the plant's size, shape, texture, and behavior give clues about its healing properties. For example, comfrey and mullein have large, lobe-shaped leaves that resemble the lungs, and they are, in fact, beneficial for the lungs. Aloe vera mends rapidly when an incision is made in a leaf, and similarly, aloe helps skin abrasions to heal quickly.

Malachite, a bright green stone, has bubbly or bull's-eye patterns. The energy of malachite seems to bubble up to the surface, often quite joyfully. Malachite is a joyful stone that helps bring emotions up to the surface.

Now close your eyes and hold the stone in the area of each of your seven major chakras. Ask for a general reading for the stone in relation to the chakras, rather than a specific reading for your personal relationship with this stone (later you can do a personal reading in a similar manner, by changing your intention). Feel how the energy of the chakra interacts (or fails to interact) with the stone. You may or may not be able to feel this. You might feel something and then your mind might say, "Oh, no, it's just my imagination." Ignore that. Pay attention to what you feel, no matter how subtle. But if you do not feel anything, don't worry. We each have different gifts, and this might not be yours. Just relax and play.

When I hold the malachite over my first and second chakras, I don't feel anything particular. Holding it over the third chakra, I feel significant movement and a sense of expansion. The third chakra relates to the emotions and personal power, so I ask my energy body whether the stone is affecting the emotions or the personal power, or both. With the malachite, it seems to be affecting the emotions.

After going through all seven chakras, bring the stone back to your third eye, where your higher intuition resides. Hold it a couple of inches in front of your forehead. Then ask the stone, "What is your healing power?" Breathe deeply and wait for an answer.

## Terminology of Stones

The stones that are used for healing may be called crystals, rocks, stones, or gemstones. Technically most rocks, trees, metals, and bones are crystals—with the exception of obsidian, because a crystal is a solidified form of a substance that has a regularly repeating arrangement of atoms resulting in natural external plane facets.

Quartz crystals are composed of silicon dioxide, and they naturally grow with points that have six external plane facets leading to a single termination. This includes clear quartz, which is translucent, meaning that light can pass through it. Milky quartz is opaque, meaning that you can't see through it. Amethyst is violet because the quartz combines with manganese to make a purple color. Rose quartz is pink, smoky quartz is brown, and citrine is yellow. The colors of quartz are caused by the mixture of elements.

Gems are cut and polished stone, and a gemstone is a mineral or crystal that has the potential to be cut and polished as a gem because of its hardness and beauty.

Cutting, grinding, and polishing stones is known as lapidary work. The scientist who studies the atomic structures within the crystal is practicing crystallography. A person who collects rocks is known as a rockhound.

You may find or buy stones that are either rough and in their natural form, or cut or tumbled by humans in a variety of shapes and sizes. They may be tumbled in a rock tumbler, which is a process similar to being rolled in a creek bed. They may be cut into various shapes to make jewel quality gemstones. The most common shape is the rounded oval cabochon. The translucent stones (gemstones) may be faceted (cut geometrically with flat plains) that enable the stone to catch light more effectively.

The tumbled or jewel quality gems are best for making tinctures and charging water, alcohol, or oil, since they have no loose particles to come out in the liquid. In healing, smooth tumbled stones are good for smoothing over rough situations. Gem quality and translucent stones help bring light into dark situations. On the other hand, rough stones penetrate to the depths and bring buried feelings to the surface.

There are human-tooled stones designed with great skill by artists who, like master sculptors, bring out the potential qualities of these stones. Many of these artists commune with the stones and know exactly how the stone wants to be cut.

If a human-hewn stone attracts you, and you feel the energy is good, then get it. But it is a good idea to cleanse it carefully, because it will hold the energy of the person who worked it. Likewise, crystals decorated with silk thread, feathers, combinations of metal, and various designs should always be purified before using, since these decorations also hold the energy of the person who worked with them. On the other hand, if you feel that person has especially good energy, you may not want to clean them.

The best guideline when buying stones is that you should have a good feeling about them. Follow your intuition and buy the first one you feel drawn to.

## Stone Kits

Before you can work with stones, you will need to have at least one stone for each chakra, and preferably more. Tiny stones don't carry much energy, so look for stones that are as big as you can afford. If your funds are limited, start with medium-sized, inexpensive, tumbled stones. You will find that even these are effective, especially when used directly on the skin (with the large stones, this is not necessary). Later when you become more familiar with the stones, you can buy larger ones. Go to a rock shop and select the stones that appeal to you, because the process of selecting each stone will be the beginning of a meaningful relationship. As you work with the rocks, you may find that you will remember exactly where you were when that rock came into your life. It is unlikely that anyone else can choose the healing rocks that will hold deep meaning for you, unless it is someone who knows and loves you, or someone who is psychically sensitive. If there is no rock shop in your area, stone kits may be available (see Resources).

## Beginner's Kit

These are the bare minimum supplies that I recommend for beginners:

- 1 single-terminated smoky quartz crystal
- 2 garnets
- 2 black obsidians
- 1 tiger's eye
- 1 carnelian
- 1 citrine
- 1 turquoise
- 1 rose quartz
- 1 B.C. jade
- 1 azurite or azurite-malachite
- 1 amethyst
- 1 large single-terminated clear quartz crystal (translucent or milky)

## Crystal Healer's Kit

If you do a few healings and it feels good, and you feel ready to make an investment in crystal healing, you will want these stones:

- 1 long thin crystal wand (at least 3 inches long and one-half inch in diameter)
- 1 large single-terminated clear quartz crystal
- 4 medium single-terminated clear quartz crystals (at least 2 inches long and one-half inch in diameter)
- 1 double-terminated clear quartz crystal
- 2 long thin delicate clear quartz crystals
- 2 single-terminated smoky quartz crystals
- 2 garnets
- 2 or 3 obsidians (at least one should be fist-sized)

2 tiger's eyes

2 carnelians

2 citrines

1 or 2 turquoise

1 or 2 malachite

2 or 3 rose quartz (at least one should be fist-sized)

1 watermelon tourmaline

2 B.C. jade (from British Columbia)

1 aventurine

1 lapis lazuli

1 azurite or azurite-malachite

2 sodalites

2 amethysts

Two stones of each type are recommended because when you do a layout, you often use two stones on either side of a central stone. For example, if a person needs more heart energy, you can put a large rose quartz at the center of the chest, with a B.C. jade on either side and two aventurines below the jades and two long thin delicate crystals between the jade and aventurine, with the terminations pointed toward the center of the chest.

The larger stones of any particular grouping are usually more powerful than the smaller ones. So a large rose quartz tends to be more powerful than a small rose quartz. But some small stones are unusually powerful. Deep rich colors bring greater intensity to a stone, as does a strong design. (In some cases, as with amethyst, pale colors also have a high value.) For example, the bull's-eye is inherent in the pattern of the malachite, and a small stone with a clearly defined bull's-eye may be more powerful than a larger, less-defined stone. You will get better results with high-quality stones that are large, with strong designs and good energy.

## Cleansing the Stones

When you use stones for healing or getting rid of negativity, it's good to clean them. There are many elaborate methods of cleansing, but I find the simplest is to hold them under cold running tap water. Since energy follows water, the undesirable energy will wash down the drain. It's also a good idea to put your hands and wrists under cold running water.

Clear quartz crystals absorb a lot of energy, so it's especially important to do this with your crystals. Hold the crystal with the termination pointing downward, toward the drain. Each stone can be washed for five to fifteen seconds or longer, according to how hard they've had to work. If you're sensitive to their energy, you'll know when they're clean. If the water gets too cold for your hands, just set them in the sink, under the flow of the tap. If you're not sensitive to the energy, give each one about fifteen seconds. If the work was very intense, give them a full minute.

When you receive a new crystal, or if your crystal has been doing especially difficult work, it's a good idea to bury it in sand, or dirt, or cover it with salt water for one to three days. Salt water can be prepared by dissolving one tablespoon of sea salt or Kosher or Hawaiian salt in one quart of warm water. Or you can use ocean water. If you don't have a yard you can keep a container of sand or dirt for burying your stones, and you can use it repeatedly, but change it periodically. For example, if you're using it for cleansing obsidian that has been used for intensive liver cleanses, you should change the sand after a few treatments. If you only use it a couple times a month for special stones, you could keep the same sand or dirt for three to six months. Sea water should be freshened every two weeks. Arrange the stones so there is at least one inch of space between each stone.

Another method is to smudge the stones with smoke from burning sage, cedar, or sweetgrass. These herbs have been used for centuries by indigenous people for eliminating negative energies. This method is especially good for stones that are decorated with feathers or metal, or that are too large or too fragile to hold under water.

## Stones as Jewelry

Stones may be worn simply for their radiant colors or great beauty, or they may be worn therapeutically. While any stone may be displayed anywhere on the body, lower chakra (first, second, and third) stones are best as bracelets, rings, belt buckles, toe rings, or anklets;

fourth and fifth chakra stones as pendants over the heart or throat; sixth and seventh chakra stones as earrings, nose rings, or tiaras. If you feel uncomfortable wearing any stone, take it off.

One story will illustrate the importance of choosing your jewelry wisely. Kathleen came to see me for a Vibrational Alignment (which includes the use of crystals) because unexplained tears that kept forming at her right eye. When we met she was wearing a diamond necklace and earrings. As usual, I asked her to remove her jewelry before the session.

As we worked it became clear that her right side (her male side) was extremely weak, even though she had a successful career. I noticed that the left side of her face looked quite handsome, strong, and relaxed, while the right looked troubled, pinched, and fearful. As I felt the spin of energy at each hip and talked about what I felt there, she revealed that she received her primary nurturing from her father, while her mother seemed emotionally distant and preoccupied.

When Kathleen turned ten years old, her period began and she started to develop breasts. Her father abruptly pulled away, which is not unusual. Many men panic when they find themselves feeling sexually attracted to their young daughters. This is tragic, especially at adolescence, when a girl's self-image may be strongly influenced by how her father reacts to her. When a father reacts as Kathleen's father did, a girl may feel shameful about her sexuality, her body, and her femininity.

At the age of ten, Kathleen was thrown back on her mother for support. Her mother resented men, and Kathleen was ripe to take on her mother's feelings. She made a decision not to trust men. Ultimately she ended up rejecting her own male side.

The energy on Kathleen's left side (her feminine side) was consistently strong and confident, while the energy on her right masculine side was unfocused and weak. Clearly, her female side was in control. Kathleen made decisions and implemented them entirely from her feminine side. Her (feminine) intuition was powerful, and her (masculine) reasoning powers were weak.

I guided Kathleen to get in touch with her male archetype (see Glossary). (This is a technique that is beyond the scope of this book to describe.) He was cold and distant. Eventually she allowed him to get in touch with his feelings, and discovered that he was holding on to a great deal of anger and resentment. It became clear that the tears that kept forming at her right eye were a direct result of the suppression of her emotions, particularly her sorrow at being abandoned by her father.

When a person is unable to express anger, she often reacts with excessive crying. Similarly, when she is not allowed to express sadness, she may react with excessive rage. I encouraged Kathleen to express emotions that she had never been allowed to express. Then she described her male self emerging from his cave, pounding his chest, and running around "like a wild Indian."

Kathleen then realized that the diamonds—which were a gift she had given herself—were a way of reinforcing her feminine image. When I suggested that she might not want to put them on again until her male side became stronger she said, "I agree. I feel so much better—so much lighter!"

I spoke to Kathleen several weeks after the treatment. Her eye had stopped tearing. As I suggested, she was now wearing carnelian (which has strong male energy) and had put away the diamonds for special occasions.

At a talk I gave about crystals at Unity Church in Santa Cruz, I mentioned that garnets are extremely stimulating and can cause a nervous reaction, particularly when worn above the solar plexus. After the presentation a woman came up and pointed to the necklace she had been wearing. It was made of chips of garnet and citrine. She told me her daughter had given it to her three months previously, and she had been wearing it ever since. During my talk she wondered if this could be the cause of the tension she had been feeling for the last three months. I said that was very likely. She took off the necklace and immediately felt better.

## Crystal Layouts

Although the stones may be placed over the clothing, they are more effective when in direct contact with the skin, especially small stones. They can be placed anywhere on or around the body, but are usually arranged over the chakras. The stones should be left in place for at least ten minutes. When a person feels the energies of the stones, you can leave them until the sensations subside.

Many people report sensations similar to those felt during acupuncture treatment (without the possible pain): energy may travel up and down the body, not necessarily where the stone is. The stone may be experienced as being large when in fact it is small (or the reverse). There may be a sensation of comfort, protection, or nurturing that seems to emanate from the crystals. The stone may seem to vibrate. Occasionally, very brief, sharp pains may seem to shoot out from the stone along specific parts of the body. The practitioner may find that some stones become very hot after being held by himself or his client or when placed on a client.

Find someone who wants to experiment with the stones. If you're giving the treatment, begin by sitting in silence alongside him, allowing your energies to become attuned to one another, to the energies of the crystals, and to Spirit. Ideally, hold a long thin clear quartz crystal with the termination pointed toward him.

If you need protection, wear an amethyst. This is advisable when you are new to the work, or when you are feeling vulnerable, or if you sense that this person's problems are very intense or likely to trigger strong feelings in you.

Now you're ready to do a layout. Try the Chakra Balance Layout. If you feel blockages, try Charging the Chakra or Cleansing the Chakra.

Feel free to move on to the next chakra while the stones are doing their work. Sometimes you can't clear the third chakra, for example, until you've worked on the fifth chakra. Try to stay with the person until you feel the obstructions easing away.

Don't be surprised if the person you are treating breaks out crying or becomes emotional. If you are not prepared to deal with this kind of reaction, do not attempt these layouts. The stones are very powerful.

When you do layouts you will be feeling for energy obstructions. You may think you need extraordinary sensitivity to feel this, but I have found that virtually everyone knows when their hand meets an energetic obstruction. When this occurs, do a layout at the chakra closest to the obstruction. Use your intuition to attune to the person and feel what she needs, and proceed as described below.

**Crystal Energization.** You can use this exercise to pull out tension and negativity from your own body and then recharge yourself with positive energy. It only takes ten minutes, and it's better than a nap or a cup of coffee.

This layout requires four single-terminated clear quartz crystals. You may substitute single-terminated amethyst or smoky quartz crystals or combine them. The amethyst is best used at the head, and the smoky at the feet. These crystals should be at least 1½ inches long, but they don't have to be special or beautiful. In fact, if you do this layout on a bed, the stones are liable to fall off and get chipped, so don't use your favorite crystals.

Each crystal should have the terminations facing outward, away from the center of the body, and be placed two to six inches from the body. Lie down on a flat surface and place crystals in the following locations:

Above the center of the top of your head
Between and below your feet
To the right of your right wrist
To the left of your left wrist

Lie in this position for about ten minutes. Be sure no one is in the "line of fire" with the terminations of the crystals. The crystals

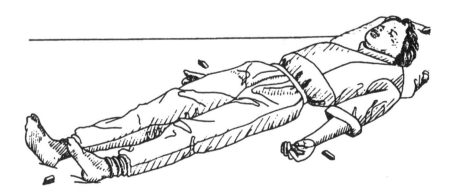

will be removing negative energy from the body and sending it out in a direct line, as if shooting out from the terminations. Anyone sitting or standing within ten feet along that line is liable to receive the negative energy.

Don't worry if you fall asleep. After ten minutes, or when the sensations subside, or when you wake up, turn each of the four crystals in the opposite direction so they are pointing toward the center of your body. Now the crystals will be charging your body with positive energy. After a few minutes try placing one or two stones on each chakra. Start out with one stone at a time, taking a few minutes to observe the energy of the stone and any changes that may take place in your energy. If you feel apprehensive while using the stones, remove them. If you don't feel anything, don't worry about it. It's a good idea to choose these extra stones before you lie down so you will have them in easy reach. After ten minutes, or when the sensations subside, remove the crystals.

**Chakra Balance Layout.** Select two stones for the first chakra to use at the groin points and one stone for each of the remaining chakras. Ask your partner to lie down, and place stones on each of the chakras. The stone at the crown chakra will lie on the table and lean against the top of her head.

Take a single-terminated clear quartz crystal, hold it in your dominant hand, and aim the point toward your partner, as you sit in silence and attune your energies. When you feel ready, hold your crystal a few inches above and pointing toward his body, beginning at the first chakra. Move your crystal very slowly two or three inches above the center of his body, from the first chakra to the crown, as you feel the energy. Ordinarily your hand will move freely, but at some point you may find that your hand slows down or simply does not want to move any farther. You may feel heat or coolness, or turbulent energy or a significant absence of energy.

Whatever chakra you are closest to when this occurs is the one that needs work. If you are in between two chakras, work on both of them. Follow the instructions on Charging the Chakra or Cleansing the Chakra, adding stones as described below.

**Charging the Chakra.** You will want to charge the chakra if energy is absent or your hand doesn't want to move past the chakra; if the energy feels cool; or if you've read the description of the chakra and believe that the energy is deficient. To charge the chakra, place one stone at the center of the area of the body corresponding to that chakra. Usually it will be a stone that corresponds to the chakra. (There are exceptions. For example, you may want to use the anti-dote—like using carnelian to close down the third eye when the energy is excessive.)

If the situation feels serious, two or three stones may be used at the center. If you're using a terminated crystal at the center of the layout (for example, a citrine crystal at the third chakra), the termination should point toward the head. Surround the central stone(s) with pairs of stones and pairs of clear quartz crystals, with the terminations pointing toward the center stone.

Leave the stones in this arrangement for at least ten minutes, or until the end of the treatment. While they are in place, encourage your partner to talk about his thoughts and feelings. Or you may feel the desire to tone. Or you may feel that it's time to move on and feel the energy at other chakras and return to this one later.

You may find yourself receiving images that you will want to share with him. Always be tentative. Say, for example, "I'm getting an image that I'd like to share with you. If it makes sense, tell me about it. If not, just let it go." Perhaps you're getting a picture of a little girl crying in a barn. Just describe what you see, without any value judgments. "I see a little girl crying in a barn. Is that familiar to you?" You may be amazed to find that when your client was four years old, her father beat her brother with a whip, and she went out to the barn to cry.

**Cleansing the Chakra.** If the energy at a chakra feels turbulent, hot, or intense, or if you've read the description for that chakra and believe that the energy is excessive, you will want to cleanse that chakra. Place a stone at the center of the area where that chakra is located. Usually it will be a stone that corresponds to that chakra, though it may be a stone from the chakra that acts as its antidote.

If you're using a terminated crystal at the center (an amethyst at the third eye for example), the termination should be pointed toward the feet to pull negative energy out of the body. Surround the center stone with pairs of crystals (these may include smoky quartz and amethyst crystals, but on the forehead they would have to be very small), with terminations pointing outward. Leave the stones in this arrangement for at least ten minutes and proceed as instructed under Charging the Chakra above.

## Correlating the Crystals with the Chakras

The following stones have been arranged according to the chakras where I most commonly use them. These are just guidelines. Any stone may be used at any chakra.

**First Chakra.** Stones for the first chakra are placed at the groin points, where the thighs join the torso, so you will need two of each stone for the first chakra.

*Red garnet* has an arousing, invigorating energy. It influences the kundalini energy that rises up the spine. Therefore it relates to the base chakra and the sixth chakra. Garnets are commonly found as small blood-colored stones. To improve fertility, place a garnet over a woman's womb a couple of inches below the naval. This is also a good placement for menstrual cramps and irregular periods.

For low back pains and premenstrual cramps, have her lie on her stomach and place a garnet at her lower back a couple of inches below the waist on the spine. This will help cleanse the blood and improve circulation. It is most effective if you use a large garnet or many small ones.

As jewelry, garnet is best worn below the waist. When above the waist, it can overstimulate the solar plexus or the pituitary in sensitive individuals, causing nervousness, headaches, or dizziness.

*Black obsidian* comes from lava that has cooled quickly. Basalt obsidian is glassy and black. This is a wonderful stone for connecting with earth energy and with your body. People who have intense emotional or spiritual experiences often find it difficult to return to the normal world, to integrate what they have experienced into their day-to-day lives. To assist these people, I place obsidian at the groin points so they won't feel too spaced out. After a healing session I give a client a big hunk of obsidian to hold. Within a few minutes the client feels grounded and can drive home safely.

I don't recommend wearing obsidian as a pendant on the chest because it prevents the easy flow of energy in and out of the heart. However, there may be times when you want to protect your heart, and wearing an obsidian over your heart is better than building walls, since it is easier to remove.

*Smoky quartz* is a brown quartz crystal that has the ability to disperse negative energies. Smoky quartz is associated with the first chakra because of its powerful connection with the earth. Though it appears to be dark, it is usually translucent when held to the light. Smoky quartz derives its dark color from exposure to natural radioactivity. Imitation smoky quartz is made by artificially radiating clear quartz. The artificially radiated stones are very dark and not translucent. I do not use them for healing.

Place the smoky quartz wherever you feel physical, emotional, or psychic blocks. Since pain is often caused by negative emotions such as resentment and anger, you can disperse pain by placing smoky quartz over the painful areas and encouraging your client to get in touch with the source of her pain.

If a client is holding on to negativity that needs to be released, lean a smoky quartz crystal against each heel, with the terminations pointing downward. This helps pull the negativity down through the feet and into the earth.

Smoky quartz is ideal for practical people: scientists, geologists, and teachers who must keep their feet on the ground but still enjoy taking excursions into the outer realms.

**Second Chakra.** These stones are orange or brown.

*Tiger's eye* connects you to the rich browns of the earth and blends with the gold of the Divine Light. You don't need to be intellectual or spiritual to enjoy the qualities of tiger's eye. Bring this stone to your third eye and it will help you see the best in everyone and feel happy about walking on the path of life. If you are in a relationship, it will help you tune into your partner telepathically.

This is a stone of courage. It gives strength and endurance and the willingness to go forward in spite of obstacles. Stroking its smooth surface will help you soothe away worries and apprehensions.

This sensuous stone is often favored as a gift between lovers. I use tiger's eye to stimulate the second chakra when a soft, gentle energy is desired. Since emotions are so connected to sexuality, thoughts about sex and love can cause anxiety and nervous tension. To calm your mind and balance your energy, hold the tiger's eye and gaze at the striped pattern, and then place (or even tape) this stone at your second chakra.

*Carnelian* is a red-orange agate that generates warmth and relaxation. It has a strong masculine energy and is good for the sexual organs, enhancing sexual energy.

Use it for tension in any part of the body, like a tiny heating pad, to bring warmth to the area, allowing the tension to ease away. Use it for tension in the shoulders and between the shoulder blades, by putting it over the tense area and even taping it in place.

You can also place carnelian over the second chakra for a sluggish digestion.

Since orange (second chakra) and indigo (sixth chakra) are antidotes, carnelian can be used when the sixth chakra has excessive energy. For example, if a person has a premature opening of the third eye, with too much psychic stimulation, place a carnelian at the third eye for just a few minutes to temporarily diminish the sixth chakra energy. Place another carnelian at the second chakra to draw the energy down and help the person come into his body.

Children are drawn to this stone. Just having a stone in their pockets will counter any tendency toward depression, negativity, or belligerence. Carnelian imparts strength, humor, and optimism.

This is the stone of worldly success. It grounds a person in the present and protects against negative energy. It will enhance self-confidence. It gives the courage to speak out. Businesspeople can wear this stone or carry it in their pockets, especially below their waists or as a ring or bracelet.

**Third Chakra.** Yellow and gold stones such as citrine and iron pyrite (so-called fool's gold) are associated with the third chakra, as are stones that have streaks or particles of copper, such as turquoise. I also put malachite at the third chakra, because it brings up the emotions, and the second and third chakras relate to the emotions.

*Citrine* is a yellow quartz that derives its color from iron oxide. Place this stone at the solar plexus to aid relaxation. It helps a person feel warmth and approval toward himself and others. Citrine puts people in touch with their personal power and encourages them to express their unique gift.

This yellow quartz aids the digestion by relaxing the organs that produce digestive juices. It frees up the breathing by relaxing the diaphragm. Use citrine to charge water and drink a few sips before each meal (see Color-Charged Water page 110).

Citrine is excellent for all mental activities. When you have difficulty concentrating or feel heavy and overwhelmed by worry and responsibilities, lie down and place one citrine on your third eye and another on your solar plexus for ten minutes while you visualize breathing in yellow light. It will help you to relax and breathe freely as it dispels negativity and gives you a more positive outlook.

Wear citrine as a pendant around your neck, preferably with the point toward your head, to improve self-confidence and feel more attuned with yourself and with Spirit. It can help break a drug habit by strengthening your self-discipline and improving your sense of self-worth.

*Turquoise* is a balancer. It opens up the heavens to the one who uses it with consciousness. It blends the color of the heavens with the color of water. It is a stone of peace, harmony, and beauty, in perfect attunement with Spirit. It is good for those who are afraid of power, or who desire to use power in a balanced way.

Turquoise is a fine stone to wear, especially set in silver. If you have digestive problems, wear turquoise as a belt buckle, bracelet, or ring. It can be worn daily to increase vitality and enhance vibratory and healing powers.

*Malachite* is a rich green stone with dark green lines that form concentric patterns like a bull's-eye. The essence of malachite is joy. Its name means emotional purger. When used over the solar plexus, malachite has the power to dredge up old buried emotional pain. It can also draw out physical pain. The larger the stone, the more powerful, though even small stones with a distinct bull's-eye pattern can be highly effective when placed directly over the painful area. Otherwise the stone should be at least as large as the area that is painful. For nausea or motion sickness, place the malachite over the solar plexus.

Malachite is good to wear as jewelry if you want to get in touch with your feelings. But if you don't want to feel vulnerable, stay away from this stone.

**Fourth Chakra.** This includes most of the pink and green stones.

*B.C. Jade* (from British Columbia) is a dark green jade that is like a loving father, reaching out his hand to give comfort, reassurance, and protection when a person feels weak and vulnerable. When the heart feels threatened or frightened, place jade directly on the heart. It has a gentle strength that is grounding and stabilizing.

Jade embodies the love of nature. It holds and gives warmth. It is soothing—especially water-worn jade. I like to carry a piece of this jade in my pocket and hold it in my hand. The stone quickly becomes warm and comforting, like holding hands with a friend.

*Green jade* is a pale green stone that is a favorite of the Chinese. They say it has wisdom, clarity, justice, courage, and modesty. It gives you the wisdom to make clear judgments, the courage to follow through on them, and keeps you from getting big-headed about the good results.

*Rose quartz* derives its pink color from titanium. It is the gentlest of stones, with a vibration that penetrates the heart, soothing away worries. For those who have been hurt in love, rose quartz is like the Divine Mother who rocks you in her arms while she exudes unconditional love. Its gentle pink ray penetrates deep into the cracks of a wounded heart. Rose quartz has the ability to heal the child within. When a person is exploring childhood traumas, place a piece at her heart.

Rose quartz is comforting for alcoholics who drink to numb the pain they feel from lack of love. Many alcoholics are highly sensitive, intuitive individuals who grew up in a society that laughed at their sensitivity. They used alcohol to dull their sensitivities. If this applies to you, and you wish to give up your dependence on alcohol, try carrying around a piece of rose quartz about the size of a quarter in your pocket. It may help alleviate your need to drink.

*Aventurine* is a light green quartz that sets up an energy that protects the heart from other people's negativity. It allows you to be soft and open without being overly vulnerable. It liberates and radiates love without being possessive. It has energy and enthusiasm. Carry it in your pocket or wear it anytime to feel a connection with its high energy.

This is the stone of the dreamer. It is helpful for those who feel too confined or inhibited; unable to break out of narrow ways of thinking. It is good for setting out on new adventures; for young people going out on their own or women going back to work after raising children.

Aventurine makes a nice present. It radiates good cheer. It is an uplifting stone that can be safely used for depression. It is delightful to wear as jewelry since it constantly gives out energy that nurtures the heart of the one who wears it as well as those who behold it.

*Watermelon tourmaline* is a beautiful green and pink stone that tends to make a person feel extremely vulnerable. It is a powerful stone to use when a client is cut off from his emotions. The green gives protection and comfort, and the pink gives vulnerability. It is like being held in loving arms that are so comforting you can no longer hold back your tears. The vulnerability that surges up with this stone can be overwhelming. The mind melts, and with it, the walls that both protect you and hold you prisoner. Don't wear this stone as jewelry unless you are prepared to be completely open-hearted.

**Fifth Chakra.** The blue stones are associated with this chakra, though lapis is also used at the sixth chakra.

*Sodalite* is a deep blue stone that often has flecks of white calcite and strongly resembles Chilean lapis. Afghan lapis, on the other hand, has unique gold flecks of iron pyrite. Sodalite can be worn safely and beneficially at all times. It will help you keep your head in the clouds and your feet on the ground.

Sodalite is invaluable for anyone having a bad drug experience, travel sickness, or depression. Hold it to your third eye and it will be your life preserver, bringing you gently back to shore.

Use this blue stone to soothe your third eye when you have been doing a lot of psychic work. Place it directly over the third eye or even tape it on. It is also useful for deepening your ability to concentrate. If you have difficulty putting your thoughts or feelings into words, or if you have stage fright, place or wear sodalite at your throat chakra, and it will help you to relax, so the words will come more easily.

Sodalite soothes all ailments of the throat. It helps reduce inflammations and swellings when used over any area of the body, provided that the stone is of at least equal size to the area that is inflamed or swollen.

*Azurite*, when used at the throat chakra, stimulates the voice box, enabling you to give voice to your thoughts and feelings. It enhances the experience and expression of your spirituality, filling you with the desire and ability to speak about deep things.

Azurite is most effective with malachite (they are often naturally combined in one stone, or two separate stones may be placed side by side). Malachite brings up buried emotions, and azurite makes a person want to talk about what he is feeling.

This stone makes beautiful jewelry. It can be worn as a necklace or earrings, to enhance spiritual awakening. It will keep you centered and articulate.

*Lapis lazuli* is a deep blue stone. The lapis found in Afghanistan is flecked with the gold of iron pyrite and often has white flecks or streaks of calcite. Chilean lapis rarely contains pyrite and is difficult to distinguish from sodalite. Afghani lapis feels more powerful.

Lapis will take you deep within the vaults of your mind. This is not a stone to use frivolously; it may be dizzying for those who are highly sensitive. When placed on the third eye, it facilitates hypnosis, visualization, astral travel, and understanding of obscure spiritual teachings. This is an excellent stone to use or to wear for ceremonial purposes.

*Sugilite* is a rich purple to violet-pink stone with streaks of black manganese. It is a rare and unusual stone, found primarily in the Kalahari region of South Africa. It is ideal for highly sensitive and gifted children—and for adults who were highly sensitive as children. It helps protect from the harshness of the world, reminding these individuals that they are special and that their gift is rare and valuable.

When discouragement or despair set in, place sugilite at the third eye, and breathe in its comforting energy. There is incredible power in a piece of good-quality sugilite, when the purple is rich and deep. It will help you believe in yourself.

This is a wonderful stone to wear as jewelry. It may make you feel as if you are on top of a mountain, with the wind blowing through your hair.

*Amethyst* ranges from deep purple to pale lavender, according to the proportion of manganese and iron in this variety of quartz. It is the gentlest of stones, yet is a powerful protector. When you wear an amethyst or keep a large cluster in a room, it has the power to allow in only those energies that are harmonious to you and to deflect and transmute other energies. It is ideal to place on your altar. Ideally, sit with the stone or cluster, hold the intent to clear the energy of the amethyst, and then hold the strong intent for it to give you protection.

Amethyst is one of the finest stones to wear, because its energy is always beneficial and protective. This stone should accompany any ceremony of protection. It can be worn when you are among people who are hostile. Hold the intention that only good energies will come to you, and all negativity will be transmuted and sent out into the cosmos as free atoms.

**Seventh Chakra.** Like brilliant stars in the sky, the clear quartz and diamonds strengthen your direct connection with Spirit. Amethyst also holds strong spiritual energy.

*Clear quartz crystals* contain the full spectrum of the energy of the seven rays. They bring more color and light into the human aura. They fill in the missing colors in the aura. When you meditate with crystals or use them for healing, they energize your chakras, burning through blocks and dispelling darkness.

When the energy of the crown is closed, put a large, single-terminated clear quartz crystal on the pillow above the center of the head, pointing away from the body. Clear quartz holds the vibration of White Light, and as you open your higher chakras you become receptive to that light and to the crystals that embody it.

When *diamonds* are energetically clean, they uplift the spirits and help a person feel good about himself, and valuable. They remind a person to be all that you can be. But when a person becomes depressed, diamonds also hold that energy and reinforce your stuck places. So instead of wearing a diamond all the time, it is preferable to remove it if you are feeling depressed.

Diamonds hold the original program they were given with, even after being cleansed. This makes them especially appropriate for marking and symbolizing occasions such as engagements and weddings. When someone gives you a diamond, be sure that you know what program it is being given with, because they come with hidden agendas. Diamonds are capable of holding these programs, just as they hold a specific resonant frequency.

One of the best ways to cleanse a diamond is to bury it in sand. This can be done each night. If a diamond has never been cleansed and if it holds negative energy, bury it in sand for a week.

Zircons have flat energy compared to true diamonds.

# Conclusion

Humankind has not woven the web of life. We are but one thread within it. Whatever we do to the web, we do to ourselves. All things are bound together. All things connect.—*Chief Seattle*

AND SO, THIS BOOK COMES TO AN END. I HOPE I HAVE INSPIRED you to take time to smell the flowers, to commune with the stones, to look up into the sky, to breathe in the colors. It is a great blessing to be walking upon this planet earth.

If we remember, each day, to give thanks to the Creator, to the earth herself, to the plant and animal and nature spirits, to our families and our beloved friends, to the water, the flowers, the trees, the sky, even the insects, the animals, and the rocks, then we begin to come into a blessed harmony with All That Is.

# Endnotes

**Introductory Material**

1. Pali Jae Lee and Koko Willis, *Tales from the Night Rainbow, Mo'olelo o na Po Makole, The Story of a Woman, a People, and an Island,* An oral history as told by Kaili'ohe Kame'ekua of Kamalo, Moloka'i 1816-1913 (Honolulu: Night Rainbow Publishing Co., 1990), 18.

2. Valerie Hunt, *Infinite Mind—Science of the Human Vibrations of Consciousness* (Malibu: Malibu Publishing, 1996), 78.

3. Herbert Benson, M.D., Julie Corliss, and Geoffrey Cowley, "Brain Check," *Newsweek,* September 27, 2004, www.msnbc.msn.com/id/6038621/site/newsweek, 2004.

**Part 1 / Vibrational Healing and the Chakras**

1. I. Prigogine and I. Stengers: *Order Out of Chaos: Man's New Dialogue with Nature* (New York: Bantam Books, 1984), quoted in Valerie Hunt, *Infinite Mind.*

2. Shirley Miekka, "Physiology of Pace," 1995, adapted from Carla Hannaford, "The Physiological Basis of Learning and Educational Kinesiology, course manual, 1992.

3. F. Batmanghelidj, M.D., *Your Body's Many Cries for Water* (Falls Church, VA: Global Health Solutions, Inc., 1997).

4. Valerie Hunt, *Infinite Mind—Science of the Human Vibrations of Consciousness* (Malibu: Malibu Publishing, 1996), 26.

5. Masaro Emoto, *The Message from Water* (Leiden, Netherlands: Hado Publishing, 1999), 18–53, 87, 89–104, 127.

6.  Fabien Maman, *The Role of Music in the Twenty-First Century* (California: Tama-Do Press, 1997), 61.

7.  Michael Talbot, interview by Jeffrey Mishlove, *Synchronicity and the Holographic Universe*, videotape (Berkeley, CA: Think Allowed Product, 1991).

8.  Deepak Chopra, MD, *Perfect Health—The Complete Mind Body Guide* (New York: Harmony Books, 1990), 12.

9.  Gary Zukav, *The Dancing Wu Li Masters—An Overview of the New Physics* (New York: William Morrow, Quill, 1979), 57.

10.  Chopra, 1990, 12.

11.  Dr. Helen Caldicott, "At the Crossroads," *New Age Magazine*, December 1977. See also National Academy of Sciences. National Research Council, *The Effects on Populations of Exposure to Low Levels of Ionizing Radiation*, Report of the Advisory Committee on the Biological Effects of Ionizing Radiations (BEIR Report), Washington, D.C., June 1976.

12.  United States Food and Drug Administration Centers for Devices and Radiological Health, "X-Rays, Pregnancy, and You," HHS Publication No. (FDA) 94-8087, www.fda.gov/cdrh/consumer/xraypreg.html.

13.  Swami K.M. Tayumanavar, personal conversation, 1989.

14.  Richard Gerber, M.D. *Vibrational Medicine—New Choices for Healing Ourselves* (Santa Fe: Bear, 1988), 128.

15.  Stanley Krippner and Daniel Rubin. *The Kirlian Aura, Photographing the Galaxies of Life,* "Bioplasma or Corona Discharge?" *in Thelma Moss and Kendall L. Johnson,* (New York: Anchor Books, 1974), 69–70.

16.  M. Alan Kazlev, "The Chakras," www.kheper.net/topic/ chakras/index.html, July 29, 2005.

17.  Manly P. Hall, *The Secret Teachings of All Ages—An Encyclopedic Outline of Masonic, Hermetic, Qabbalistic and Rosicrucian Symbolical Philosophy* (Los Angeles: Philosophical Research Society, 1988), CXXXVII.

18.  C.W. Leadbeater, *The Chakras* (Wheaton, Il.: Quest, Theosophical Publishing, 1977), 18–21.

19.  Bill Moyers, *Healing and The Mind,* "The Chemical Communicators" by Candace Pert (New York: Doubleday, 1993), 179–180.

20. Marc Carlson, "Historical Witch Trial Stats (Revised)," 1998, www. malaspina.com/burning/burnwit6.htm.

21. Kyla Ward, "The Inquisition, Witch is Witch," first appeared in *Tabula Rasa #1*, 1994, www.tabula-rasa.info/DarkAges/Inquisition.html.

22. "Health and Medicine in Medieval England," May 2002, www. historylearningsite.co.uk/health_and_medicine_in_medieval_.htm.

23. Kazlev, *The Chakras*.

24. A major source of contention involves the so-called spleen or splenic chakra. According to M. Alan Kazlev, based on information from Alfred Ballabene, the idea of the spleen chakra came from Alice Bailey, the Theosophist who channeled a source she called "The Tibetan." Through both her and Leadbeater, the second chakra became known as the spleen or splenic chakra.

25. C.W. Leadbeater, 1977, 41.

26. Kazlev, "The Chakras."

27. Sri Aurobindo, *Letters on Yoga, vol. I* (Twin Lakes,WI: Lotus Press, 3rd ed., 1995), 27–28.

28. Kazlev, "The Chakras."

29. Olga Kharitidi, *Entering the Circle: Ancient Secrets of Siberian Wisdom Discovered by a Russian Psychiatrist* (Albuquerque: Gloria Press, 1995), 221–226.

30. Personal conversation with Hopi Spokesman David Monongye in Hotevila, Arizona in 1967.

31. Frank Waters, *Book of the Hopi* (New York: The Viking Press, 1965), 9–12.

32. Kazlev, "The Chakras."

33. Caroline Myss, *Sacred Contract: Awakening Your Divine Potential* (New York: Random House, 2002), 166–168.

34. Barbara Ann Brennan, *Hands of Light: A Guide to Healing Through the Human Energy Field* (New York: Bantam Books, 1988), 46.

35. Hunt, 1996, 29.

36. Leadbeater, 1992, x, 1, 4, 5, 7.

37. Valerie Hunt, "Sound Therapy and the Human Energy Field," Fifth International Sound Colloquium (Loveland, CO: August 14–17, 1997).

38. W. Brugh Joy, *Joy's Way* (Los Angeles: J.Tarcher, 1979), 155–156.

39. Shafica Karagulla, *Breakthrough to Creativity* (Marina Del Ray, CA: DeVorss, 1967), 61.

40. Hunt, 1996, 11, 19, 21.

41. Ibid., 18, 19, 21, 27.

42. Ibid., 14-16.

43. Itzhak Bentov, personal communication with Richard Gerber in 1977, quoted in Gerber, *Vibrational Medicine*, 133.

44. Michael Talbot, *The Holographic Universe* (New York: Harper Collins, 1991), 97, 140.

45. Ibid., 97.

46. Ibid., 184.


Part 2 / Light, Color, and Frequencies

1. Frank Waters, *Book of the Hopi* (New York: Viking Press, 1965), 8.

2. NASA, "Imagine the Universe! Electromagnetic Spectrum, Introduction," http://imagine.gsfc.nasa.gov/docs/science/know.11emspectrum. html.

3. Berkeley Lab, "Micro Worlds: Exploring the Structure of Materials, Electromagnetic Radiation," www.lbl.gov/MicroWorlds/ALSTool/EMSpec/ EMSpec.html.

4. John Ott, *Health and Light*, (New York: Pocket Books, 1976), 34.

5. World Health Organization (WHO), "What Are Electromagnetic Fields?" www.who.int/peh-emf/about/WhatisEMF/en/.

6. Albert Roy Davis and Walter C. Rawls, *Magnetism and its Effects on the Living System*, (New York: Exposition Press, 1974), 6–7.

7. Hunt, 1996, 30–31.

8. Matthew J. Parry-Hill et al, "Basic Electromagnetic Wave Properties," National High Magnetic Field Laboratory, Florida State University, http://micro.magnet.fsu.edu/prmer/java/wavebasics, August 18, 2004.

9.  Dictionary Labor Law Talk.com, "Definition of Color," http:// encyclopedia.laborlawtalk.com/colors.

10. Gary Zukav, *The Dancing Wu Li Masters—An Overview of the New Physics* (New York: William Morrow, 1979), 51.

11. Robert L. Lehrman, *Physics The Easy Way, Second Edition* (Hauppauge, NY: Barron's Educational Series, Inc., 1990), 296–297.

12. Matthew J. Parry-Hill and Michael W. Davidson, "Interactive Java Tutorials, Primary Additive Colors," www.micro.magnet.fsu.edu/primer/java/ primarycolors/additiveprimaries/, August 13, 2004.

13. Mark Wieczorek, "Color Theory," www.marktaw.com/design/Color Theorya.html, Oct 05, 2004.

14. NASA, "Electromagnetic Spectrum," http://son.nasa.gov/content/ electrospectrum.htm.

15. Association of Teachers' Websites, "Gondar Design Science," http:// imagine.gsfc.nasa.gov/docs/science/ know_11/emspectrum.html. See also NASA "Imagine the Universe!–Electromagnetic Spectrum– Introduction," http://imagine.gsfc.nasa.gov/docs/science/know_11/ emspectrum.html, and Lehrman, 1990, 298.

16. Environmental Services and Consultation Oregon Health Services, Office of Environmental Toxicology, Dave Stone, "Ultraviolet Light Germ Transmission Demonstrations," www.dhs.state.or.us/publichealth/esc/ docs/uvlight.cfm. See also John Ott, 1976, 38.

17. NASA, "Imagine the Universe!" website.

18. NASA, "Imagine the Universe!" website.

19. Hunt, 1996, 19.

20. Berkeley Lab website.

21. Lehrman, 1990, 289.

22. Ellen O'Connor, "Psychological Studies in Nonionizing Electromagnetic Energy Research," *Journal of General Psychology,* January 1993.

23. University of California, Davis, Environmental Health & Safety, "Radiological Safety," http://ehs.ucdavis.edu/hp/shi/index.cfm. See also NASA, "Imagine the Universe!" website.

24. ATW website, "Gondar Design Science." See also NASA, "Imagine the Universe!" website.

25. Russ Rowlett and the University of North Carolina at Chapel Hill, "How Many? A Dictionary of Units of Measurement," www.unc.edu/~rowlett/units.

26. International Institute of Biophysics, The German Research Groups, Neuss, Germany, "Who We Are and What We Do," www.lifescientists.de/ib0200e_.htm, 2003. See also Popp, F.A., "Experimental Investigations on Ultraweak Photon Emission From Biological Systems," ed. Eric P., and P. Schram, Proceedings Internation Symposium on Analytical Applications of Bioluminescence and Chemilumiscence, Brüssel, 1978, 601–617, and Popp, F.A., "Biophotons and Their Regulatory Role in Cells," *Frontier Perspectives*, The Center for Frontier Sciences, Temple University, Philadelphia, 7, 1998, 13–22.

27. Michael Talbot, *The Holographic Universe* (New York: Harper Collins, 1991), 27.

28. Intelegen, Inc., "What is the Function of the Various Brainwaves?", www.brain.web-us.com/brainwavesfunction.htm, 2003.

29. The Monroe Institute, "What are Binaural Beats," www.monroeinstitute.org/research/hemisync/binaural.html, accessed January 17, 2005.

30. Center for Neuroacoustic Research, "Epsilon, Gamma, HyperGamma and Lambda Brainwave Activity and Ecstatic States of Consciousness," c. 1999, www.jeffthompson.com/registry/articles/articleepsi.htm.

31. Hunt, 1996, 63–64. See also Crawford 2000, "Geophysical Condition: Earth's Rising Base Frequency," www.crawford2000.co.uk/sch2htm, and David Jordan, "The Earth's Frequency," www.geocities.com/davidjay jordan/EarthsFrequency.html.

32. Nick Anthony Fiorenza, "Planetary Harmonics in Light, Sound, & Brain Wave Frequencies," http://lunarplanner.com/Harmonics/planetary harmonics.html, June 29, 2003. See also Richard Alan Miller and Iona Miller, "The Schumann Resonances and Human Psychobiology," *Nexus Magazine*, 10, 3 April-May 2003, www.nexusmagazine.com/articles/schumann.html.

33. Hunt, 1996, 19, 21.

34. Author's communication with Bruce Tainio (September 2004) who attributes this information to Dr. Fritz Popp, Ph.D., German biophysicist and professor.

35. Young, D. Gary, N.D., *Aromatherapy, the Essential Beginning* (Essential Press Publishing, 1996), 38, 40. Young's book used Hz measurement but Bruce Tainio (see reference 34) states that the correct measurement is MHz.

36. Tim Wilson, "Chant: The Healing Power of Voice and Ear, An Interview with Alfred Tomatis, M.D.," in *Music: Physician for Times to Come, An Anthology*, compiled by Don Campbell (Wheaton, IL: Quest Books, 1991), 13, 17.

37. Robert L. Lehrman, *Physics The Easy Way, Second Edition* (Hauppauge, NY: Barron's Educational Series, Inc., 1990), 167.

38. John C. Lilly, *The Mind of the Dolphin, A Nonhuman Intelligence*, http://eccosys.jp/lilly/dolphinMind03.html.

39. J. Stone, "Why do cats purr?" *Scientific American*, September 16, 2004, www.sciam.com/askexpert.

40. Clifford L. Laurence, *The Laser Book—A New Technology of Light* (New York: Prentice Hall, 1986), 9.

41. John Ott, 1976, 7.

42. Laurence, 1986, 4, 6, 9.

43. Ibid., 6.

44. Ibid., 2, 5.

45. Lehrman, 1990, 294.

46. Laurence, 1986, 2–5.

47. Wilson, 1991, 19–25. See also Jacob Liberman, O.D. Ph.D., *Light—Medicine of the Future* (Santa Fe: Bear, 1991), 91.

48. Ibid., 30–33.

49. Walter Pierpaoli, "Melatonin Extends Rat Lives," *Brain/Mind Bulletin* 13, no. 9 (June 1988), 1, 8.

50. Dr. Glen M. Swartwout, *Color & Light* (Pahoa, HI: Remission Foundation Trust), 1.

51. R. Relkin, "Miscellaneous Effects of the Pineal," in *The Pineal Gland*, ed. R. Relkin (New York: Elsevier Biomed, 1978), 247–272. See also H. Samis et al, "Aging and Temporal Organization," in *Interventions in Aging*, ed. R. Walker and R. Cooper (New York: Marcel Dekker, Inc., 1983), 397–419.

52. J.N. Ott, "Color and Light: Their Effects on Plants, Animals, and People," *Journal of Biosocial Research* 7, part I (1985).

53. A. Fisher, "Light: Nature's Mysterious Essential Gift," *Geo Magazine* 3, (Oct, 1981), 66–78.

54. Liberman, 1991, 51.

55. Melyni Worth, PhD., "Low Level Laser Therapy Provides New Treatment Possibilities," *World Equine Veterinary Review* 9, no. 3 (1998).

56. John Ott, 1976, 30–33.

57. Ibid., 48–49.

58. Ibid., 57–69.

59. Ibid., 61.

60. Ibid., 150.

61. Ibid., 55.

62. Ibid., 70–71.

63. Ibid., 72–73.

64. Ibid., 193–194.

65. Ibid., 196.

66. Ibid., 9.

67. Liberman, 1991, 153.

68. Ibid, 43–44.

69. Ibid., 45–46.

70. John Ott, 1976, 54–55.

71. Swartwout, 8.

72. John Ott, 1976, 192–193.

73. Liberman, 1991, 151.

74. Ibid., 60.

75. The Orchid House, "Some Data on Commonly Available Fluorescent Tubes," http://retirees.uwaterloo.ca/~jerry/orchids/tubes.html.

76. John Ott, 1976, 192–193.

77. Liberman, 1991, 61.

78. V. Beral et al, "Malignant Melanoma and Exposure to Fluorescent Light at Work," *Lancet* 2 (1982): 290–292.

79. John Ott, 1976, 148.

80. Swartwout, 20.

81. John Ott, 1976, 116.

82. Ibid., 161–162.

83. Swartwout, 21.

84. Liberman, 1991, 154.

85. John Ott, 1976, 110–111.

86. Liberman, 1991, 59.

## Part 3 / Healing with Color (Chromotherapy)

1. *Paul Cezanne: The Man and the Mountain*, video, a Glashaus Film Production in association with RM Arts, 1985.

2. Dr. Laing, author's Spirit Guide, received 1976, Eugene, Oregon.

3. Robert Lawlor, *Voices of the First Day—Awakening in the Aboriginal Dreamtime* (Rochester, VT: Inner Traditions, 1991), 114–116.

4. Manly P. Hall, *The Secret Teachings of All Ages* (Los Angeles: Philosophical Research Society, 1988), CXXXIX.

5. Health Research, *Color Healing, An Exhaustive Survey Compiled from 21 Works of Leading Practitioners of Chromotherapy* (Mokelumne Hills, CA: Health Research, 1956), 1–34.

6. Helen Graham, *Discover Color Therapy* (Berkeley: Ulysses Press, 1998).

7. Darius Dinshaw, *Let There Be Light* (Malaga, NJ: Dinshaw Health Society, 2003), 14.

8. Ibid., 7–8.

9. Teresa E. Quinlan, M.D., personal communication with the author, Columbus, Ohio, May 2003.

10. Liberman, 1991, 188–189.

11. Jan Turner and Lars Hode, *Low Level Laser Therapy* (Grangesberg, Sweden: Prima Books, 1999), 21.

12. Melyni Worth, Ph.D., "Low Level Laser Therapy Provides New Treatment Possibilities," *World Equine Veterinary Review*, 3, no. 3 (1998).

13. Turner and Hode, 1999.

14. Joy Gardner, *The Book of Guidance* (Winlaw, B.C.: Healing Yourself Press, 1985), 18–19.

### Part 4 / Healing with the Voice

1. Hazrat Inayat Khan, *The Mysticism of Music, Sound and Word, The Sufi Message, Volume II* (Delhi: Motilal Banarsidass, 1988), 157–158.

2. Deepak Chopra, MD, *Perfect Health, The Complete Mind/Body Guide* (New York: Harmony Books,1990), 131–133.

3. Frank Waters, *The Book of the Hopi* (New York: Penguin Books,1977), 3–5.

4. William K. Powers, *Sacred Language; The Nature of Super-natural Discourse in Lakota* (Norman, OK: University of Oklahoma Press, 1986), 154.

5. Ibid., 57, 82, 60.

6. Joseph Epes Brown, *The Sacred Pipe, Black Elk's Account of the Seven Rites of the Oglala Sioux* (Norman, OK: University of Oklahoma Press, 1971), 45.

7. Ibid., 67–100.

8. Robert Lawlor, *Voices of the First Day—Awakening in the Aboriginal Dreamtime* (Rochester, VT: Inner Traditions, 1991), 184–193.

9. Pamela Amoss, *Coast Salish Spirit Dancing, The Survival of an Ancestral Religion* (Seattle: University of Washington Press, 1978), 52–54, 142.

10. Ibid., 161, 127–129.

11. Susan Wallenberg, personal conversation, Fairfax, California, June 1992.

12. Powers, 1986, 70.

13. Lawlor, 1991, 180.

14. Lance, "Hail to the Sabbat," www.paganet.org/pnn/v10/i3/sabbat.html.

15. "Chakra Vortex of Light—Sounds of the Chakras," www.nettally.com/krivera/sound.html, 2004.

16. Max Freedom Long, *The Secret Science Behind Miracles* (Marina del Rey, CA: DeVorss & Co., 1976), 191–193.

17. Marlo Morgan, *Mutant Message Down Under* (New York: Harper Collins, 1994), 92.

18. Long, 1976, 193.

19. Dan Campbell, *The Mozart Effect* (New York: Avon Books, 1997), 23.

20. Joy Gardner, *Healing Yourself During Pregnancy* (Berkeley, CA: Crossing Press, 1987), 22–23.

21. John Ortiz, Ph.D., "Sound Psychology: the Tao of Music," *Positive Health Magazine*, www.positivehealth.com/permit/Articles/Sound_and_Music/ortiz29.htm.

22. J.W. and J. M. Standley, "The Effects of Music Listening on Physiological Responses of Premature Infants in the NICU," *Journal of Music Therapy*, 32 (1995): 208–227.

23. E. M. Buday, "The Effects of Signed and Spoken Words Taught with Music on Sign and Speech Imitation by Children with Autism, *Journal of Music Therapy*, 32 (1994): 189.

24. D. L. Nelson, V. G. Anderson, and A.D.Gonzales, "Music Activities As Therapy for Children with Autism and Other Pervasive Developmental Disorders," *Journal of Music Therapy*, 21 (1984): 100–116.

25. L.L. Morton, J.R. Kershner, and L.S. Siegel, "The Potential for Therapeutic Applications of Music On Problems Related To Memory and Attention," *Journal of Music Therapy*, 27 (1990): 195–208.

26. D.M. Ricks and L. Wing, "Language, Communication, and the Use of Symbols In Normal and Autistic Children," *Journal of Autism and Childhood Schizophrenia*, 5 (1975): 119–221.

27. M.A. Wooten, "The Effects of Heavy Metal Music on Affect Shifts of Adolescents in an Inpatient Psychiatric Setting," *Music Therapy Perspectives* 10, 1992, 93–98.

28. L.M. Bailey, "Music Therapy In Pain Management," *Journal of Pain and Symptom Management* 1 (1986): 25–28. See also S.L. Beck, "The Therapeutic Use of Music for Cancer-Related Pain," *Oncology Nursing Forum*, 18 (1991): 1327–1337. See also H.M. Heckman and J.B. Hertel, "Pain Attenuating Effects of Preferred Versus Non-Preferred Music Interventions," *Psychology of Music* 21 (1993): 163–173.

29. Mitchell L. Gaynor, M.D., *Sounds of Healing–A Physician Reveals the Therapeutic Power of Sound, Voice, and Music* (New York: Broadway Books, 1999), 14–16.

30. Jim Oliver, notes from CD: *Harmonic Resonance* (New York: The Relaxation Company, 1995).

31. Karen Allen, PhD et al, "Normalization of Hypertensive Responses During Ambulatory Surgical Stress by Preoperative Music," *Psychosomatic Medicine*, 63 (2001): 487–492, www.psychosomaticmedicine.org/cgi/content/full/63/3/487.

32. Dale Bartlett, Donald Kaufman, and Roger Smeltekop, "The Effects of Music Listening and Perceived Sensory Experiences on the Immune System as Measured by Interleukin-1 and Cortisol," *Journal of Music Therapy* 30 (1993): 194–209.

33. Susan Aldridge, PhD, "Music with Exercise Boosts the Brain," Heart and Circulation Center, www.healthandage.com.

34. T.K. Cordobes, "Group Songwriting as a Method for Developing Group Cohesion for HIV-Seropositive Adult Patients with Depression," *Journal of Music Therapy* 34 (1997): 46–67. See also G. Wijzenbeek, and N. van Nieuwenhuijzen, "Receptive Music Therapy with Depressive and Neurotic Patients," *Music Therapy and Music Education for the Handicapped* (St. Louis: MMB Music, Inc., 1993), 175.

35. S. Boldt, "The Effects of Music Therapy on Motivation, Psychological Well-Being, Physical Comfort, and Exercise Endurance of Bone Marrow

Transplant Patients," *Journal of Music Therapy* 33 (1996): 164–188. See also J.M. Standley, "Music Research in Medical/Dental Treatment: Meta-analysis and Clinical Applications," *Journal of Music Therapy* 23 (1986): 56–122.

36. Bradford S. Weeks, MD, "The Physician, The Ear and Sacred Music," *Music Physician for Times to Come, An Anthology* compiled by Don Campbell (Wheaton, IL: Quest Books, 1991), 41.

37. Tim Wilson, "Chant: The Healing Power of Voice and Ear; an interview with Alfred Tomatis, MD," in *Music Physician for Times to Come,* 13, 17.

38. Michael Moore, *Fahrenheit 9/11* (video documentary), Dog Eat Dog Films, June 25, 2004. See also Bloodhound Gang, "The Roof is on Fire Lyrics," www.sing365.com/music/lyric.nsf/The-Roof-is-on-Fire-lyrics-Bloodhound-Gang/4B8AFCFD3214FA7548256D250006E497, January, 2005.

39. Don Campbell, 1997, 53.

40. Alfred Tomatis, *The Conscious Ear* (New York: Station Hill Press, 1991), 125.

41. Don Campbell, 1997, 15.

42. Ibid., 50.

43. Weeks, 1991, 19, 13–14.

44. Ibid., 47

45. Wilson, 1991, 13,17.

46. Ibid., 18–21, 23.

47. Marla Jo Fisher, "Joy of singing in a choir could be preventive medicine, researchers say," *Knight Ridder/Boston Globe*, March 31, 2001, 5.

48. Howard Richman, "The Entrainment Transformation Principle," www.soundfeelings.com/products/alternative_medicine/music_therapy/entrainment.htm, October 16, 2004.

49. Laurel Elisabeth Keyes, *Toning, The Creative Power of the Voice* (Marina del Rey, CA: DeVorss & Co., 1973), 99.

50. Shark exhibit at Monterrey Bay Aquarium in Monterrey, CA, November 1991.

51. Keyes, 1973, 99–100.

52. Barry Lynes, *Dr. Royal Rife, The Cancer Cure that Worked—50 Years of Suppression,* (Queensville, Ont: Marcus Books, 1987).

53. Kay Gardner, *Sounding the Inner Landscape: Music as Medicine* (Stonington, ME: Caduceus Publications, 1990), 29. See also B.M. Stone Clinic, "What is Lithotripsy," www.geocities.com/HotSprings/Villa/5556/lith. htm., January 9, 2005.

54. *The Varieties of Healing Experience: Exploring Psychic Phenomena in Healing.* Transcript of Interdisciplinary Symposium of October 30, 1971. Academy of Parapsychology and Medicine, Los Altos, CA: 1973.

55. "Principles of Underwater Sound, Chapter 8," *Fundamentals of Naval Weapons Systems,* www.fas.org/man/dod101/navy/docs/fun/part08.htm. See also National Academy of Sciences, "Beyond Discovery, The Path from Research to Human Benefit," *Sounding Out the Ocean's Secrets,* www2.nas.edu/bsi

56. John Kehe, "Navy Sonar Threatens Marine Mammals," www. newconnexion.net/article/07-01/sonar.html.

57. Keyes, 1973, 108.

58. Norman Cousins, *Anatomy of an Illness* (New York: Bantam Books, 1991), 30–43.

59. Gaynor, 1999, 46–50.

60. Dr. H. Spencer Lewis, *Sanctum Invocation and Vowel Intonations,* a cassette tape from record S-33, Rosicrucian Supply Bureau.

61. Joy Gardner-Gordon, *The Healing Voice—Traditional and Contemporary Toning,Chanting and Singing* (Freedom, CA.: Crossing Press, 1993), 102–103.

62. Ibid., 100.

63. Barbara Marciniak, *Bringers of the Dawn,* (Rochester, VT: Inner Traditions/Bear, 1992), 192–197.

64. Wilson, 1991, 19, 25.

**Part 5 / Healing with Aromatherapy**

1. Tom Robbins, *Jitterbug Perfume* (New York: Bantam Books, 1990), 228.

2. Shirley Price, *The Aromatherapy Workbook* (San Francisco: Thorsons/ HarperCollins, 1993), 1.

3. D. Gary Young, N.D., *Aromatherapy: The Essential Beginning* (Salt Lake City: Essential Press, 1996), 8–10.

4. Price, 1993, 2.

5. Patricia Davis, *Aromatherapy—An A-Z* (Saffron Walden: C.W. Daniel, 1988), 7.

6. Young, 1996, 1, 9, 44. See also Price, 1993, 16.

7. Young, 1996, 16.

8. Jean Valnet, MD, *The Practice of Aromatherapy* (Rochester, VT: Healing Arts Press, 1990), 28.

9. Davis, 1988, 3–5.

10. Price, 1993, 7.

11. Young, 1996, 17. See also Davis, 1988, 8.

12. Davis, 1988, 8.

13. Young, 1996, 17–18.

14. Price, 1993, 9.

15. Young, 1996, 2–5.

16. Price, 1993, 2–3.

17. Renata Nummela Caine and Geoffrey Caine, "Making Connections: Teaching and the Human Brain (Nashville, TN: Incentive Publications, 1990), www.buffalostate.edu/orgs/bcp/brainbasics/triune.html. See also "Brain Function and Physiology," www.brainplace.com/bp/brainsystem/ limbic.asp, January 14, 2005.

18. Young, 1996, 22.

19. Henry Gray, *Anatomy of the Human Body* 14th ed., (New York: Barnes & Noble, 1995), 720.

20. Young, 1996, 23.

21. Valnet, 1990, 69.

22. Ibid., 69–71.

23. S. Zhao, "Scientific Research of Essential Oils at Weber State University," presented at Young Living Essential Oil Conference, 1996.

24. Young, 1996, 29–30.

25. Valerie Worwood, *The Fragrant Mind,* (Novato, CA: New World Library, 1996), 3.

26. Rev. Marcy Foley, N.D., *Embraced by the Esssence!—Your Journey Into Wellness Using Pure Quality Essential Oils* (Eldridge, IA: Bawden Printing, 1998), 26.

27. Kathi Keville and Mindy Green, *Aromatherapy: A Complete Guide to the Healing Art* (Berkeley, CA: Crossing Press, 1995).

28. Dr. Light Miller and Dr. Bryan Miller, *Ayurveda and Aromatherapy* (Twin Lakes, WI: Lotus, 1995), 84–91.

29. Valnet, 1990, 73.

30. Bruce Tainio in personal conversation with the author, November, 2003.

31. Malcolm Dixon and Edwin C. Webb, *Enzymes* (New York: Academic Press, 1964), 794–808.

32. Bruce Tainio in personal conversation with the author, November, 2003.

33. Young, 1996, 40. Young's book used Hz as a measurement, but Tainio states (see endnote 32) that the correct measurement is MHz.

34. Infinity Resources FAQ. See also Young, 1996, 38. Young's book used Hz as a measurement, but Tainio states that the correct measurement is MHz.

35. Foley, 24

36. Young. 1996, 38. Young's book used Hz as a measurement, but Tainio states that the correct measurement is MHz. See also Infinity Resources FAQ.

37. Barry Lynes, *Dr. Royal Rife: The Cancer Cure That Worked—50 Years of Suppression* (Queensville, Ont: Marcus Books,1987).

38. Foley, 27.

39. Young, 1996, 20.

40. Valnet, 1990, 27.

41. Young, 1996, 8–9.

42. Price, 1993, 15–16.

43. Young, 1996, 48–49.

44. Ibid., 51.

45. Ibid., 52.

46. Price, 1993, 16.

47. Ibid., 20–21.

48. Susan Renkel, R.N., "What is CO2 Extraction," 1998, www.naturesgift. com/CO2.htm.

49. Daniel Penuel, M.D., *Natural Home Health Care and Essential Oils* (Hurricane, UT: Essential Science Publishing, 1998), inside front cover.

50. Davis, 1988, 7.

51. Young, 1996, 27.

52. Ibid., 27.

53. Sandra Richardson, "Essential Oils: Nature's Perfect Solutions," www.vibrantoils.com, 2003.

54. Angela Rosa, R.N., *Aromatherapy: Medicinal and Energetic Use of Plant Essences* (Hawi, HI: Essential Health, 2003), 12.

55. Valerie Worwood, *The Fragrant Mind* (Navato, CA: New World Library, 1996), 221–226.

56. Rosa, 2003, 23.

57. Ibid., 7.

## Part 6 / Healing with Crystals

1. Melissa Applegate, "The Legacy of Marcel Vogel," the transcript of a paper presented at the 1996 2nd Annual Advanced Water Sciences Symposium, www.vogelcrystals.net, 1996-2004.

2. Frank Waters, *Book of the Hopi* (New York: Viking Press, 1965), 11.

3. John Kaimikaua, talk at Molokai, HI: 1997.

4. Rita H. Delorme, "Ring of the Lord: The Ring of Bishop Francis X. Gartland Still Inspires," Archives of the Catholic Diocese of Savannah, Georgia, www.diosav.org/News/NewsIndex.asp?Criteria=Article& SelectedID=264&CategoryID=16.

5. Anselmus De Boot, *Gemmarum et lapidum historia,* liber. I, caput 26, Lugduno, Batava, (University of Leiden, Netherlands: 1636), 103.

6. George Frederick Kunz, Ph.D., *The Curious Lore of Precious Stone* (New York: Dover Publications, Inc., 1971), 23.

7. Ibid., 24.

8. Science Museum of Virginia website: www.smv.org/prog/xtaldsc/htm.

9. Melody, *Love Is In the Earth: a Kaleidoscope of Crystals, Updated* (Wheat Ridge, CO: Earth-Love Publishing, 1995), 31.

10. Science Museum of Virginia website, "Introducing Crystals," www.smv. org/prog/xtaldsc.htm.

11. William Peez, *Crystals in the World Around Us,* www.yale.edu/ynhti/ curriculum/units/1989/6/89.06.06.x.html.

12. Richard Gerber, M.D., *Vibrational Medicine* (Santa Fe, NM: Bear, 1988), 337–338.

13. Ibid., 326.

14. Ibid., 327.

15. Jeff Tyson, "How LCDs Work," 2005, www.electronics.howstuffworks. com/lcd1.htm.

16. Science Museum of Virginia, "Introducing Crystals," www.smv.org/prog/ xtaldsc.htm.

17. R. Miller, "The Healing Magic of Crystals: An Interview with Marcel Vogel," *Science of Mind,* August, 1984.

18. Gerber, 364-365.

19. Michael Talbot, *Synchronicity and the Holographic Universe,* video (Berkeley, CA: Thinking Allowed Productions), an interview by Jeffrey Mishlove, 1991).

20. "Are Near Death Experiences Real?" www.mikepettigrew. com/afterlife/ html/history_of_ndes.html.

21. Grof, Stanislav and Christina, "Experiences of Clinical Death and Near-Death," www.sju.edu/cas/theology/Courses/1141/Shamansim/grof.htm.

# Glossary

**allopathic:** A method of treating disease by the use of agents that produce effects different from those of the disease treated (as opposed to *homeopathic*).

**antidote:** An antidote counteracts the effect of a substance, as hot antidotes cold and cold antidotes hot. See page 97 for instructions on how to use antidotes for color and chakra healing.

**archetype:** In Jungian psychology, an inherited unconscious idea universally present in individual psyches.

**aromatherapy:** A form of therapy that uses the aromas of plants for medicinal purposes. This is usually done in the form of essential oils derived from flowers.

**carrier:** A carrier carries essential oil onto the skin. It is usually a cold pressed vegetable, seed, or nut oil such as almond or mild sesame oil. Jojoba is a liquid wax that works well as a carrier because it does not go rancid.

**chakra:** A Sanskrit word that means wheel. It is used to describe the spinning energy in the energy field, primarily in the vicinity of the spine. Technically *chakrum* is the singular term for which *chakra* is plural, but in the west the word *chakra* is used for both. Sometimes it is spelled *cakra*.

**chakra diagnosis:** A method of retrieving information about the body, mind, emotions, and spirit by feeling the spin of energy at each of the seven chakras along the spine to form a coherent picture of the whole person. (See also "Chakra Diagnosis" on page 33.)

**chromotherapy:** The use of color and light to gently bring about homeostasis. Colored light is applied to specific areas on the body.

**clairvoyant:** Having the paranormal ability to see energies and objects or actions beyond the range of natural vision.

**coherent:** Anything that is highly organized.

**complementary medicine:** A group of diverse medical and health care systems, practices and products not presently considered part of conventional (allopathic) medicine, when used in combination with conventional medicine.

**entrainment:** The tendency for two oscillating bodies to lock into phase so that they vibrate in harmony.

**flower remedies:** The Bach Flower Remedies originated with Dr. Edward Bach, a homeopath who lived in London in the early 1900s. He induced in himself various mental and physical imbalances. Then he wandered about, looking for the right flowers to balance his energies. He collected, named, and described thirty-eight remedies that became known as the Bach Flower Remedies. Since then, many gifted people have tuned into the flowers in their bioregions and have produced a wide variety of excellent flower remedies or essences.

**fundamental tone:** The root of a chord in music—the lowest note in a series of harmonics.

**harmonic:** A single oscillation whose frequency is an integral multiple of the fundamental frequency. Harmonics are a series of oscillations in which each oscillation has a frequency that is an integral multiple of the same basic frequency.

**homeopathy:** A form of medicine that uses preparations chosen according to the principle of "let like be treated by like." For example, epilepsy (a convulsive disease) may be treated by a plant that, in large doses, produces convulsions. A minute amount of this plant is combined with a larger amount of inert material (such as alcohol), and is then triturated (rubbed down) or percussed (shaken vigorously) so that the two substances are finely mixed. This produces a potentized vibrational remedy, which has a more powerful curative reaction in the body than a greater quantity of the original crude substance, and yet it is harmless. For example, homeopathic poison ivy may be taken internally to treat an allergy to poison ivy. Potencies are designated according to the decimal scale. Higher potencies are vibrationally stronger, though they contain increasingly less of the original substance. Many homeopaths are also doctors.

**ions:** Charged particles in the air that are formed in nature when enough energy acts upon a molecule such as carbon dioxide, oxygen, water, or nitrogen to eject an electron from the molecule leaving a positively charged ion. The displaced electron attaches itself to a nearby molecule, which then becomes a negatively charged ion. Negatively charged ions of oxygen (negative ions) inhibit the growth and reproduction of airborne pathogens and increase the human sense of well-being. They can be found abundantly in nature by waterfalls, on the beach, and in the mountains. They can also be generated by brushing hair.

**Kahuna:** A Hawaiian priest and healer who usually specializes in a particular area such as herbology or chanting.

**Kirlian photography:** A technique invented by Russians Semyon and Valentina Kirlian that makes use of high-voltage spark discharges to provide a picture of the energy fields.

**kundalini:** Energy that lies dormant at the base of the spine until it is awakened by yoga or other spiritual disciplines, and channeled upward through the chakras in the process of spiritual perfection. *Premature kundalini rising* or *spiritual emergency* occurs when the energy goes up the spine before a person is properly prepared, sometimes getting stuck at undeveloped chakras, causing physical or emotional symptoms that can be extremely uncomfortable or disconcerting.

**melody:** A sequence of single tones, usually in the same key or mode, to produce a rhythmic whole—often a tune, air, or song.

**naturopathy:** A form of healing performed by a naturopath. A Naturopathic Doctor (N.D.) receives similar training to that of a Medical Doctor (M.D.), but the medicines used are natural, including fasting, special diets, herbal and homeopathic remedies, and acupuncture.

**neet:** Undiluted oils that are not mixed with a carrier.

**negative ions:** See ions.

**octave:** A Western octave consists of eight notes and twelve semitones. The eighth full note above a given tone, having twice as many vibrations per second, or below a given tone, having half as many vibrations per second. An octave is equal to 130.8 Hertz. The Indian octave or *saptak* consists of seven notes and is divided into twenty-two intervals.

**overtones:** Any of the higher tones heard with a fundamental tone, having a frequency or vibration that is an exact multiple of the frequency of the fundamental tone. Vocal overtones can be deliberately created by adjusting the jaw and altering the mouth cavities.

**pendulum:** An object that is suspended from a fixed point that moves back and forth freely. A hanging ornament or necklace. Pendants or necklaces in which the ornament is symmetrical can be used as a pendulum. A crystal is often suspended from a chain and used as a pendulum.

**piezoelectric effect** (pronounced pie-ee'-zo): A measurable electrical voltage produced when mechanical pressure is applied to quartz crystals. An actual spark may be emitted.

**pitch:** The number of vibrations per unit of time, which creates a low (slow vibrations) or high (fast vibrations) sound. Pitch refers to setting the key of the voice or a musical instrument in a particular vibrational frequency.

**Reiki:** A Japanese form of laying-on-of-hands brought to the United States in 1938 by Mrs. Hawayo Takata (1900–1980). My teacher, Bethal Phaigh, received transmission directly from Mrs. Takata. I was initiated in Second Degree Reiki by Bethal in 1982.

**resonance:** The reinforcement and prolongation of a sound or musical tone by reflection or by sympathetic vibration of other bodies.

**rhythm:** Rhythm gives definition, pattern, and boundary to the tone. It can be a consistent repetitious beat or completely spontaneous, moving in and out of a beat pattern. Rhythmic patterns can be constant, syncopated or completely chaotic.

**sound healing:** (Not defined in the current dictionary.) The therapeutic application of sound frequencies to the body/mind of a person with the intention of bringing them into a state of harmony and health.

**sounding:** (This usage is not given in the current dictionary.) Making spontaneous and/or uninhibited sounds without specific melody, rhythm or words, though melody, rhythm, and words may emerge spontaneously.

**tantra:** Form of yoga described in comparatively recent Hindu or Buddhist religious writings concerning mysticism and magic. Some of these writings describe methods of rechanneling sexual energy. Many modern New Age teachers use these and other techniques for raising or spiritualizing the sexual energy.

**Theosophists:** Adherents of a modern mystical religious movement that originated in the United States in 1875 around the teachings of Madame Helena Blavatsky and Alice Bailey, who were influenced by Buddhist and Brahmanic theories, especially of pantheistic evolution and reincarnation.

**tone:** The utterance of a sound that is distinct and identifiable by its regularity of vibration, or *constant pitch* (as distinguished from noise), so that it may be put into harmonic relation with other such sounds or instruments or voices.

**toning:** The use of sustained vocal tones, usually vowel sounds, without melody, rhythm, or words, usually made on the exhalation of the breath.

**velocity:** The speed at which a wave travels.

**Vibrational Alignment™:** A method of Vibrational Healing originated and taught by Joy Gardner that combines chakra diagnosis with vibratory tools to balance the energy of body, mind, spirit, and emotions.

**Vibrational Healing or Medicine:** Vibrational Healing acknowledges that we are all vibrations, and that when this universal energy is in balance we are in a state of health. When it is blocked or out of balance illness tends to occur. Vibrational Healing attempts to bring physical, emotional, mental, and spiritual energies into alignment by focusing sound, light, color, gemstones, aromatic oils, and other vibratory tools where they are needed.

**vibratory tools:** Healing tools that have a strong, unique frequency that interacts with the human energy field. These tools include light, color, crystals, aromatherapy, sound, flower remedies, gem elixirs, homeopathy, and others.

**volume:** The intensity of sound and the fullness of tone. The loudness of a sound corresponds to the amplitude of the wave.

**Wheatstone bridge:** British physicist Charles Wheatstone (1802–1875) was responsible for popularizing the arrangement of a simple mechanical instrument consisting of a circuit with two pairs of resistors, connected in a loop, with a battery and a galvanometer linking the junction between one pair and the other. Bridges are among the most accurate types of measuring devices used to determine the value of an unknown resistance when the other three resistances are known.

# Recommended Reading

## On Aromatherapy

Maury, Marguerite. *Marguerite Maury's Guide to Aromatherapy*. Saffron, Walden: The C.W. Daniel, 1990.

Price, Shirley. *The Aromatherapy Workbook*. San Francisco: Thorsons/ Harper-Collins, 1993.

Valnet, Jean, MD. *The Practice of Aromatherapy*. Rochester, VT: The Healing Arts Press, 1990.

Young, D. Gary, N.D. *Aromatherapy: The Essential Beginning*. Salt Lake City: Essential Press,1996.

## On the Chakras

Brennan, Barbara Ann. *Hands of Light—A Guide to Healing Through the Human Energy Field*. New York: Bantam Books, 1988.

Bruyere, Rosalyn. *Wheels of Light: Chakras, Auras, and the Healing Energy of the Body*. New York: Simon and Schuster/Fireside, 1994.

Gardner-Gordon, Joy. *Pocket Guide to Chakras*. Berkeley, CA: Crossing Press, 1998.

Judith, Anodea. *Wheels of Life—A User's Guide to the Chakra System*. St. Paul: Llewelllyn Publications, 1996.

Myss, Caroline. *Energy Anatomy*. Louisville, CO: Sounds True, 2002. (12 cassettes)

## On Color and Light

Dinshah, Darius. *Let There Be Light. Light*. Malaga, NJ: Dinshah Health Society, 2003.

Gaynor, Mitchell L., M.D. *Sounds of Healing: A Physician Reveals the Therapeutic Power of Sound, Voice, and Music.* New York: Broadway Books, 1999.

Graham, Helen. *Discover Color Therapy.* Berkeley, CA: Ulysses Press, 1998.

Liberman, Jacob, O.D., Ph.D. *Light—Medicine of the Future.* Santa Fe: Bear & Company, 1991.

Ott, John. *Health and Light.* New York: Pocket Books, 1976.


**On Crystals**

Gardner, Joy. *Color and Crystals: A Journey Through the Chakras.* Berkeley, CA: The Crossing Press.

Melody. *Love Is In the Earth: A Kaleidoscope of Crystals, Updated.* Wheat Ridge, CO: Earth-Love Publishing House, 1995.

Raphaell, Katrina. *Crystal Enlightenment.* Santa Fe: Aurora Press, 1986.

Richardson, Wally and Huett, Lenora. *Spiritual Value of Gemstones.* Marina del Rey, CA: DeVorss, 1983.


**On Toning**

Campbell, Don G. *The Roar of Silence.* Wheaton, IL: Theosophical Publishing House, 1989.

Gardner-Gordon, Joy. *The Healing Voice: Traditional and Contemporary Toning, Chanting, and Singing.* Berkeley, CA: The Crossing Press, 1993.

Goldman, Jonathan. *Healing Sounds: the Power of Harmonics.* Rockport, MA: Element, 1992.

Goldman, Jonathan. *Shifting Frequencies.* Flagstaff, AZ: Light Technology Publications, 1998.

Keyes, Laurel Elizabeth. *Toning, The Creative Power of the Voice.* Marina del Rey, CA: DeVorss, 1984.

Tomatis, Alfred. *The Conscious Ear.* Station Hill Press, 1991.

*Music: Physician for Times to Come, An Anthology* compiled by Don Campbell. Wheaton, IL: Quest Books, 1991.

**On Vibrational Healing**

Gerber, Richard, M.D. *Vibrational Medicine—New Choices for Healing Ourselves.* Santa Fe: Bear, 1988.

Hunt, Valerie. *Infinite Mind—Science of the Human Vibrations of Consciousness.* Malibu: Malibu Publishing, 1996.

# Resources

### Altered States of Planet Earth CD
My own CD of shamanic sounding accompanied by musician Alejo playing the didjeridoo. Excellent for massage, trance dancing, and entering altered states. See www.joy.highvibrations.net.

### BT3 Frequency Monitoring System
This machine developed by Bruce Tainio may be seen at www.tainio.com.

### Certified Vibrational Healers
Joy's website at www.joy.highvibrations.net carries information about Certified Vibrational Healers in various locations.

### Colored Lamp and Filters (Gels)
A simple lamp that takes plastic gels is carried by Vita-Gem Enterprises (www.vitagem.com). Darius Dinshah recommends using high-quality plastic theatrical filters. These thin plastic gels cost a fraction as much as the glass sheets. He recommends Roscolene Filters, which can be ordered from Samarco Inc., P.O. Box 153008, Dallas, TX 75315-3008, phone 214-421-0757. At the time Dinshah's book was published (2003), the numbers that corresponded to the recommended colors were as follows: red 818, orange 809 & 828, yellow 809, lemon 809 & 871, green 871, turquoise 861 & 871, blue 859 & 866, indigo 828 & 859 & 866, violet 832 & 859 & 866, purple 832 & 866, magenta 818 & 828 & 866, scarlet 810 & 818 & 861. When two or three numbers are used for one color, combine all of those filters (one on top of the other) in any order. Because the colors and numbers sometimes change, when you contact Samarco, tell them you want the colors that Dinshah recommends. Dinshah advises that when you order the filters, make sure that the numbers agree with the above list and carefully mark each one with its number. Disregard the theatrical names given to the colors. Already assembled filter sets are available in 6½ by 6½

inches or 8 by 10 inches. If you are using the lamp from Vita-Gem, you need to specify to Samarco that the film size should be 6½ by 7¾ inches.

## Handheld Healing Lasers

High-quality lasers combine colored light diodes, infrared light, and a multiple range of frequencies from 1 to 20,000 Hertz. You can learn more about low level laser therapy (LLLT) and high-quality handheld healing lasers from: www. Quantum-Healing-Lasers.com. You can get a five percent discount if you mention this book.

## Healing Stones by Joy Gardner

In my lapidary studio I work with healing stones, shaping them from rough rock into the exact shapes and sizes that the stones themselves want. Some of these can be viewed through my website at www.joy. highvibrations.net. Special orders are taken for stones that you need, or you may have your own raw materials that you want shaped or repaired. Prepackaged stone kits may be available. Email me at vibes@aloha.net.

## The Healing Voice—Toning the Chakras

My cassette tape guides you through color breathing and toning for each of the chakras. See www.joy.highvibrations.net.

## Joy Gardner's Vibrational Healing Program

I have been teaching this program since 1989. Currently it is structured as a four-week program, taught in two segments over a one-year period, with four experiential workshops per two-week segment. The workshops promote profound personal healing, deep inner growth, increased self-confidence, following your Inner Voice, and finding your Divine Purpose. Because these attributes are an essential part of a full and self-realized life, many of my students come simply for their own healing or for their own personal development. The required reading ensures that all students will begin with a common body of knowledge, so that students at all levels of expertise may be taught simultaneously. Graduates of the program may attain certification as Vibrational Healers. Currently the workshops included in the curriculum are: The Healing Voice; Emotional Release; Balancing the Chakras with Gemstones; Aromatherapy and Sound; Underlying Cause—the Roots of Disease; Core Belief Work; Past Life Regressions; Intuition, Meditation and Releasing Earthbound Spirits; Chakra Diagnosis and Vibrational Alignment™. For information about the Vibrational Healing Program and other talks and workshops see www.joy. highvibrations.net.

## Joy Gardner's Website

Please see www.joy.highvibrations.net for more than a hundred pages of information about the Vibrational Healing Program, magazine articles, certified vibrational healers, a newsletter, excerpts from my books and samples from my tape and CD.

## Cynthia Mitchell, Sound Healer

Cynthia describes her work as "providing a landscape of sound that a person can rest in." For more information see my website at www.joy.highvibrations.net/joy/practitioners.html.

## Seed Sounds

Harish Johari, a North Indian musician, composer, poet, artist, and Tantric scholar, has produced a tape of the traditional Vedic "Sounds of the Chakras." It is available at www.tantra.com/tantra2/30-040.html.

# Index

abdominal breathing, 152–153
absolutes, 191, 194
additive color system, 61
adrenal cortex, 183
Akashic Records, 71–72
Allen, Karen, 137–138
alpha waves, 69, 71
*Altered States of Planet Earth* (CD by Joy
    Gardner), 151
amethyst, 211, 215–216, 228, 229, 239
amplitude, 57, 58
amygdala, 180–181
*Anatomy of an Illness* (Cousins), 151–152
Anderson, Alan F., 90
Anderson, Mary, 31, 32
angelica essential oil, 198, 201
antidotes, 97-98, 109, 231
Apache sounding ceremony, 129–134
aphrodisiac, 175, 202
Arderne, John, 15
*Aromatherapie (The Practice of Aroma-*
    *therapy)* (Valnet), 177, 183
aromatherapy
    chakra-oil correlation, 202–206
    effectiveness of, 173
    healing with essential oils, 201–202
    history of, 174–178
    Joy Gardner's experience with,
        188–191
    practical aspects of, 191–201
    science of, 180–188
    spiritual/magical uses of, 178–180
aromatic water, 193
"The Art of Medicine" (Arderne), 15
Ashoka (Buddhist king), 174
aspirin, 29

*Atlantic Medical Journal*, 102
audible sounds, 73–74
auras, 7, 11, 23-24, 72, 95–97, 201–202
Aurobindo, Sri, 17
Australian Aborigines, 119, 122–124,
    126, 128–129
Avalon, Arthur (John Woodroffe), 16, 19
Avicenna (Arab physician), 99, 176
Ayurvedic medicine, 120

Babbit, Edwin, 100
bacteria, 176, 183–185
Baldwin, Kate W., 102
base notes, 192
bath oils/salts, 199
B. C. jade, 236
Beck, Robert, 70, 71, 142
becquerel, 56
Bekesy, Georg von, 67–68
Belaiche, Paul, 177–178
Beltane, 127
Bentov, Itzhak, 27–28
Besant, Annie, 15
beta waves, 69
Bible, 117, 174–176, 179–180
biological frequencies, spectrum of,
    65–78
Bird, Christopher, 208
black obsidian, 45, 232–233
Blascovich, K., 137
Blavatsky, Madame, 15
blockages, xiv
blood pressure, 137–138
bloodstone, 211
blue, 97, 97–98, 100, 111, 113, 205,
    237–239

273

essential oils, 40, 72–3. *See also*
    aromatherapy
eucalyptus oil, 183, 205
expression, 193–194
extraction, 191–195
eyeglasses, 91–93
eyes, 91–93, 111, 196

face, color healing for, 111
Farag, Dr., 184
father, 35, 38, 47, 226
Father C. R. C., 12
Feingold, Ben F., 86
female archetype, 226
fertility, 126-127
fifth chakra, 23, 36, 48–49, 98, 111, 205,
    237–239
first chakra, 23, 35, 47, 97–98, 202,
    232–233
fluorescent bulbs, 89-91
foods, 72, 86, 114–115, 187
Fourier, Jean Baptiste Joseph, 67
Fourier transforms, 67
fourth chakra, 23, 36, 97, 108, 204,
    236–237
Four Worlds, 120–121
*The Fragrant Mind* (Worwood), 201
France, aromatherapy in, 176,
    177–178
frankincense oil, 175-176, 206
Fredericks, Oswald White Bear,
    18–19
frequencies
    anatomical/food, 72–73
    brain frequencies, 69–72
    of crystals, 213
    crystals, pattern alteration, 214
    electromagnetism, 51–65
    of essential oils, 173, 186–188
    Hertz frequencies, 55–56
    high frequency sounds, 140
    of invisible light, 61–63
    of light bulbs, 89
    music, effects of, 142
    resonance, entrainment, 143–144
    of sounds, 73–74
    spectrum of biological, 65–78
    of visible light, 58–61
    wavelength, 56–58
full-spectrum light, 79–87, 90, 94

Gabby, Samuel Lee, 85
gamma brain waves, 70
gamma-rays, 65
Gardner, Joy
    chakras, experience with, 30–33
    crystals, experience with, 215–218
    essential oils, experience with, 188–191
    healing effects of music, 135–136
    journey of, xix-xxii
    sounding, experience with, 129–134
    spectrum of biological frequencies,
        65–78
    toning experiences of, 150–151
Garfield, Laeh Maggie, 150
garnets, 227, 232
Gattefossé, René-Maurice, 177
Gaynor, Mitch, 135, 154
gem, 221
gemstones, 221. *See also* crystals, healing
    with
geranium, 202
Gerard, Robert, 88
Gerber, Richard, xxii
German chamomile, 205
Ghadiali, Dinshah P., 100–101
Gichtel, Johann Georg, 12–13, 14
glass, 103, 104, 105
Golden, Lawrence, 137–138
Goswami, Shyam Sundar, 17
Graves' Disease, 7–10
Greeks, 176, 212
green, 111, 113, 236–237
green jade, 236
Green, Mindy, 184–185
Gregorian chants, 141–142
Gregory (pope), 141
groaning exercise, 163–164
group toning, 167–171

Ha'a lelea Kawaia'a, Raylene, 210
*Hands of Light* (Brennan), 20, 29
harmony, 144–146, 167-168
Hawaiians, 121, 127–128, 129, 209–210
healer, Vibrational Healer, 11
*Healing Vacations in Hawai'i, A Travel
    Guide to Retreats, Alternative Healers
    and Spas* (Sims), 45
*The Healing Voice* (Gardner), 162–163
*Healing Yourself During Pregnancy*
    (Gardner), 134

*Healing Yourself* (Gardner), xix
*Health and Light* (Ott), 79, 82–83
heart, 65, 137–138, 139, 204. *See also*
    fourth chakra
Heim, Albert von st. Gallen, 217
Helmholtz, Hermann von, 67
Hemi-Sync, 70
herbs, 177, 190, 225
Herschel, William, 62
Hertz frequencies
    brain frequencies, 69–72
    colors of light measured with, 59–60
    measurement of, 55–56, 65
    measurement of sound, light in, 58
    resonance, 143–144
    smell measurement in, 67
    Spectrum of Biological Frequencies
        and, 68
Hertz, Heinrich Rudolf, 56
Hesychastic tradition, 17-18
high-intensity discharge lamps (HID), 89
Hills, Christopher, 32
hippocampus, 180–181
Hohenheim, Theophrastus Bombastus
    von (Philippus Aureolus Paracelsus),
    99–100
Hollwich, Fritz, 90-91
Holographic Body Assessment, 33–34
*The Holographic Universe* (Talbot), 4
home, 74, 112–113
Hopi Indians, 18–19, 51, 120–121, 209
Horn Chips, 121–122
Huichol Indians, 118
human body
    bodily harmony, 144–146
    brain frequencies, 69–72
    electromagnetism, 54–55
    frequency of, 187–188
    light/color, practical applications of,
        87–94
    light, response to, 80, 81–82, 85–87
    toning for pain in, 164–165
    vibrations, effects of, 64
Hunt, Valerie
    altered state research, 24–27
    aura frequency, 72
    on colors of chakras, 20–21, 22
    diagnosis of field disturbances, xv
    electromagnetism experiments by,
        54–55

measurement of energy fields, 1–2
on mystics, frequency, 71
use of microwaves, 64
Huygens, Christian, 142
IBM, 207
illness, 72, 97, 157, 183–191
Imhotep, 174
Inayat Khan, Hazrat, 117
incandescent bulbs, 89
indigo, 98, 111
*Infinite Mind, Science of the Human
    Vibrations of Consciousness* (Hunt), xv,
    24–25
infrared light, 62, 80, 107, 184
International Enzyme Commission, 186
invisible light, 61–63
invocation, 42–43

Jesus Christ, 18
jewelry, 225–227
*Jitterbug Perfume* (Robbins), 173
Johari, Harish, 127
*Journal of the American Medical
    Association*, 137
Joy, W. Brugh, 22
Jue, Ronald Wong, 33–34

Kablaya (holy man), 122
*kahuna*, 127–128, 129, 210
Kaimikaua, John, 210
Kamehameha III (king of Hawaii), 210
Karagulla, Shafica, 22
Kazlev, M. Alan, 16
Keville, Cathy, 184–185
Keyes, Laurel Elizabeth, 151
Kharitidi, Olga, 18
Kirlian photography, xv, 11
Kirlian, Semyon and Valentina, 11
Kootenay Mountains (British Columbia),
    216–217
Krakov, S. V., 87
Krine, Zane, 93
Kubler-Ross, Elisabeth, xx, xxi, xxii,
    159–160
Kunz, George Frederick, 211

Laing, Dr., 30-31, 98, 111
Laing, R. D., 31
Lakota Indians, sound rituals of, 121–122
lambda brain wave states, 70

lamp, colored, 104
Lang, William, 31
lapis lazuli, 210, 211, 237, 238–239
Lapraz, Jean Claude, 177–178, 184
lasers, 74–78
laser therapy, low level, 107
laughter, toning with, 151-152
lavender oil, 183, 190, 193, 201, 206
Lawlor, Robert, 122–123, 126
*Layayoga—an Advanced Method of Concentration* (Goswami), 17
Leadbeater, C. W., 15–17, 21
lemon oil, 183, 204
*Let There Be Light* (Dinshah), 101-102
LFAS (Low Frequency Active Sonar), 147–148
Liberman, Jacob, 80, 87, 93, 105–107
light
  cellular response to, 78–87
  colored light, effects of, 95–97
  color/light healing techniques, equipment, 100–115
  electromagnetic wave and, 57–58
  frequencies of, 73
  invisible light, 61–63
  lasers, 74–78
  light bulbs, 89–91
  measurement of, 58
  practical applications of, 87–94
  Spectrum of Biological Frequencies, 65–74
  sunglasses, eyeglasses and, 91–93
  ultraviolet light, suntan lotion and, 93–94
  visible light, frequencies of colors, 58–61
*Light—Medicine of the Future* (Liberman), 80, 87
light box, 103–104
light bulbs, 89–91, 104
lightning, 70–71
limbic system, 180–181
Little Joe, 129–131, 133
Long, Max Freedom, 127–128, 129
Low Frequency Active Sonar (LFAS), 147–148

Maclaine, Shirley, xxi
MacLean, Paul, 180–182

Maestroni, Georges, 78–79
malachite, 210, 211, 220, 235–236, 238
male archetype, 226–227
Maman, Fabien, 2–3
Mandel, Peter, 105
Manners, Peter Guy, 144–145
Marciniak, Barbara, 167–168
massage, 165–167, 198–199
Maury, Marguerite, 178
Maypole Dance, 127
McDaniel, Karen, 135–136
Megahertz, 187
melatonin, 78–79, 90
*The Message from Water* (Emoto), 2, 208
Michigan State University, 138
microwaves, 63–64
millimeter waves, 63–64
Mitchell, Cynthia, 139
Mitchell, Edgar, 208
moaning exercise, 163–164
Monroe Institute (Faber, Virginia), 70
Morgan, Marlo, 128–129
mother, 35, 38, 47, 226
Motoyama, Hiroshi, 27–28
Mozart, Amadeus, 140
*The Mozart Effect* (Campbell), 140–141
mullein oil, 190
music, 2–3, 73, 134–142, 160–161
*Mutant Message Down Under* (Morgan), 128–129
Myss, Caroline, 19

nanometers, 58, 59
National Bureau of Standards, 71
nature, 1, 113–114
neocortex, 181
neonatal jaundice, 88
neroli, 203
nerves, of olfactory system, 181
nervous system, 105–107, 140, 205–206
neutrino, 28–29
*Newsweek*, xvi
New Testament, 175–176
*Nuclear Evolution* (Hills), 32

Oak Ridge National Laboratories, 213
obsidian, 45, 232–233
Ohio State University, 138
oils. *See* essential oils
Oldfield, Harry, 201–202

Schumann Resonances, 71
Schumann, W. O., 71
Schweitzer, Albert, 92
second chakra, 23, 35, 47–48, 98,
  108–109, 110, 111, 202–203,
  233–234
*The Secret Life of Plants* (Tompkins and
  Bird), 208
*The Secret Science Behind Miracles* (Long),
  127–128
*Secrets of Life* (Walt Disney), 80–81
seed sounds, 126–127
selects, 194
senses, 67–68, 173. *See also* aromatherapy;
  color healing (chromotherapy);
  sound healing
sensual oils, 199
*The Serpent Power* (Avalon), 16, 17, 19
seventh chakra, 23, 36, 206, 239–240
sexuality, 126–127, 183, 234
Shanti Nilaya, xx
Shoshone, 118
Sims, Susanne, 45
sixth chakra, 23, 36, 98, 108, 205, 234,
  237
skin, 195–199, 227
skin cancer, 93
smell, 67. *See also* aromatherapy
smoky quartz, 233
sodalite, 238
solvent extraction, 194
sonar, 146–148
song
  effects of, 139, 141–142
  power of sound, 117–119
  in sounding ceremony, 130, 131, 133,
    134
  in Yuwipi healing ritual, 121–122
*Song of Solomon* (Old Testament),
  174–175
soothing sounds, 156
sound, 44, 58, 73–74, 142–146
Sound Healer, 155-157
sound healing
  cultural/spiritual uses of sound,
    120–129
  power of sound, 117–119
  sounding, Joy Gardner's experience
    with, 129–134
  sound, science, medicine, 134–148

toning, 148–157
toning, emotional release through,
  157–171
toning for chakras, 171–172
sounding, 120, 129–134. *See also* toning
*Sound Physician* (Garfield), 150
Sound Surveillance System (SOSUS),
  147
Spectro-Chrome System, 101–103
Spectrum of Biological Frequencies,
  65–74
spin, 34–38, 40, 46–49
Spirit Dance, 124
Spitler, Harry Riley, 105
*Stalking the Wild Pendulum* (Bentov),
  27–28
Steiner, Rudolf, 15, 100
Steno, Nicolaus, 212
Sternheimer, Joel, 2–3
still, 176, 192
stone kits, 222–224
stones, 32-33. *See also* crystals, healing
  with
subtractive color system, 61
sun, 54
Sun Dance, 122, 126
sunglasses, 91–93
*Sunlight* (Krine), 93
sunscreen, 93–94
Swartwout, Glen, 90, 92
syntonics, 105–107

Tainio, Bruce, 67, 72, 186–187
*Take Off Your Glasses and See* (Liberman),
  93
Talbot, Michael, 4
*Tales from the Night Rainbow* (Lee and
  Koko), xiii
*The Tao of Music* (Ortiz), 134
Tayumanavar, Swami, 217–218
telemetry, 25–27
thalamus, 181
*Theosophia Practica* (Gichtel), 12–13
Theosophical Society, 15–16, 31
theta waves, 69, 71
"thieves' oil", 176
third chakra, 23, 35–36, 108, 139, 189,
  203–204, 220, 235–236
third eye, 238, 239
Thoth, 99

thought, 207–208
throat chakra. *See* fifth chakra
Tibetan Buddhism (Vajrayana Buddhism), 12
Tibetans, 154
Tiger Balm, 189
tiger's eye, 233–234
Tiller, William, 145–146, 214
time, 217
Tomatis, Alfred, 73, 139–140, 141–142, 171
Tompkins, Peter, 208
tones, 40, 109, 144–146
tongues, speaking in, 124–126
toning
  abdominal breathing, 152–153
  for chakras, 171–172
  definition of, 120
  description of, 148–150
  emotional release through, 157–171
  healing through, 136
  healthy waveforms with, 146
  instructions for, 153–157
  Joy Gardner's experience with, 150–151
  with laughter, 151–152
  prayer and, 121
  Toning for the Chakras, 171–172
*Toning, The Creative Power of the Voice* (Keyes), 151
top note, 192
totals, 195
tourmaline, watermelon, 237
turquoise, 235
Tutankhamon (pharaoh of Egypt), 174
Tyndale, John, 184

ultraviolet (UV) light
  categories of, 63
  cellular response to, 81
  description of, 62
  light bulbs and, 89
  sunglasses and, 91
  suntan lotion and, 93–94
University of Cairo, 184
U.S. Navy, 146, 147–148

Vajrayana Buddhism (Tibetan Buddhism), 12
Vallette, C., 183

Valnet, Jean, 177, 182–183, 185–186
Vibrational Alignment, 38–50
Vibrational Healing
  chakra diagnosis, 33–38
  chakras, history/locations/numbers, 12–20
  chakras, human energy field, 6–10
  chakras, science of, 24–28
  colors of chakras, 20–22
  healer, 11
  introduction to, xvii–xviii
  Joy Gardner's journey and, xxi–xxii
  music, healing effects of, 134–142
  Rainbow System, 22-24
  reasons for, 5–6
  resonance, entrainment, 142–144
  Spectrum of Biological Frequencies, 68–74
  Vibrational Alignment, 38–50
*Vibrational Healing through the Chakras* (Gardner), xiii–xxii
*Vibrational Medicine* (Gerber), xxii
vibrations, 51–65, 67–68, 142–146, 148–157. *See also* frequencies
violet, 59–60, 61, 98, 111
visible light, 58–61
Vision Quest, 121–122
visualization, 108–110
Vogel, Marcel, 207–208, 214
voice. *See* sound healing
*Voices of Ancestors* (Ywahoo), 150
*Voices of the First Day* (Lawlor), 122–123

Wagner, Richard, 112
Walt Disney, 80–81
Warburg, Otto, 184
water, 1, 2, 110–111, 208
Waters, Frank, 18-19, 120–121
Wauters, Ambika, 32
waveforms, 67, 68, 145–146
wavelength, 56–59, 61–63, 69, 77
waves, xvii–xviii, 52–58, 63–65
Webb, Edwin C., 186
Weber University, 183
websites, 58, 186
whales, 146–148
wintergreen oil, 189
Woodroffe, John (Arthur Avalon), 16, 19
word, 117, 119

Printed in the United States
by Baker & Taylor Publisher Services